Living Well Emotionally

Living Well Emotionally

Break Through
to a Life of Happiness

MONTEL WILLIAMS

with William Doyle

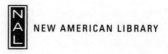

New American Library
Published by New American Library, a division of
Penguin Group (USA) Inc., 375 Hudson Street,
New York, New York 10014, USA
Penguin Group (Canada), 90 Eglinton Avenue East, Suite 700, Toronto,
Ontario M4P 2Y3, Canada (a division of Pearson Penguin Canada Inc.)
Penguin Books Ltd., 80 Strand, London WC2R 0RL, England
Penguin Ireland, 25 St. Stephen's Green, Dublin 2,
Ireland (a division of Penguin Books Ltd.)
Penguin Group (Australia), 250 Camberwell Road, Camberwell, Victoria 3124,
Australia (a division of Pearson Australia Group Pty. Ltd.)
Penguin Books India Pvt. Ltd., 11 Community Centre, Panchsheel Park,
New Delhi - 110 017, India
Penguin Group (NZ), 67 Apollo Drive, Rosedale, North Shore 0632,
New Zealand (a division of Pearson New Zealand Ltd.)
Penguin Books (South Africa) (Pty.) Ltd., 24 Sturdee Avenue,
Rosebank, Johannesburg 2196, South Africa

Penguin Books Ltd., Registered Offices:
80 Strand, London WC2R 0RL, England

First published by New American Library,
a division of Penguin Group (USA) Inc.

First Printing, January 2009
10   9   8   7   6   5   4   3   2   1

Copyright © Mountain Movers, Inc., 2009
All rights reserved

 REGISTERED TRADEMARK—MARCA REGISTRADA

LIBRARY OF CONGRESS CATALOGING-IN-PUBLICATION DATA:
Williams, Montel.
Living well emotionally: break through to a life of happiness/Montel Williams with William Doyle.
    p.   cm.
Includes bibliographical references.
ISBN 978-0-451-22664-8
1. Conduct of life. 2. Happiness. 3. Self-care, Health—Popular works. I. Doyle, William, 1957– II. Title.
BF637.C5W535 2009
158—dc22   2008044840

Printed in the United States of America

This book is dedicated to my wife, Tara,
for her endless and unwavering support.

Acknowledgments

I'd like to thank everyone who made this book possible, especially: my coauthor William Doyle, Tracy Bernstein, Melanie McLaughlin, Christine McQuaid, Mel Berger, Richard Rosenthal, Keith McLaughlin, David Smith, Sonja Lyubomirsky, Christopher Peterson, Mihaly Csikszentmihalyi, Martin Seligman, Jerome Wakefield, Allan Horwitz, Joseph Glenmullen, John Ratey, Robert Thayer, James Blumenthal, Joseph Hibbeln, Harold Koenig and David Meyers.

Contents

A Note to the Reader

Living Well Emotionally

Introduction

This book is about your happiness: how to understand it, how to cultivate it, and how to achieve it in your life.

I wrote this book because I am an expert on what depression and sadness feel like. You may be, too; you may feel overwhelmed or helpless, and you may have no one to turn to who understands your suffering.

Then I wrote this book for you. I've learned some amazing things about happiness that I want to share with you.

If you're not depressed, but you're just interested in the idea of being happier, I wrote this book for you, too.

The world is filled with narratives of personal depression. Many of these books have a common theme: depression really, really hurts. And there are countless books on happiness, too. But in this book I'm going to focus *specifically on what you can do to reduce your sadness and/or depression and increase your happiness over the long term*—based on my experience, based on the greatest wisdom of the ages, and based on the latest, most exciting medical and scientific breakthroughs.

In researching this book, my coauthor, Bill Doyle, and I reviewed three thousand years of human thought on human happiness, including the ancient Greek and Roman thinkers, Hebrew, Hindu, and Buddhist texts, the New Testament, the Koran, and the writings of the great minds of literature and psychology.

We reached out and picked the brains of some of the greatest research scientists, medical doctors, psychologists, and psychiatrists in the world today, including experts working in two exciting new fields: "happiness research" and "positive psychology." We read hundreds of their most fascinating research reports and we discussed their findings with them.

And I have some wonderful news for you.

There are paths that you and I can take that can bring us through the forest of depression and sadness, and lead us toward the sunlit fields of emotional well-being, happiness, and joy.

I will take you on a journey to the brightest and darkest places of my life, and my experiences with happiness, anger, achievements, crises, depression, drugs, and therapy.

I will take you on a Journey of the Mind, a tour of the Emotional State of the Union today: America's happiness, depression, medication, therapies, and trends, the big issues and controversies, and the best medical and scientific expert opinions.

I will take you on a Journey of the Body: the quest for emotional wellness through physical joy and the exciting new developments suggesting how exercise and diet can affect and improve emotional well-being, by elevating mood; by reducing stress, anxiety, and depression; and by increasing physical and emotional happiness.

And I will take you on a Journey of the Soul: the quest for spiritual happiness and how spiritual religious well-being is intertwined with emotional health.

Finally, I will tie it all together with the Living Well Emotionally Well-Being Program, a comprehensive program of insights, options, exercises, and ideas for achieving true joy and lasting emotional health.

In the course of my life, I have learned seven interrelated insights that changed my life for the better, and I believe they can change yours, too:

7 Insights for
Living Well Emotionally

1. You own the definition of you, and you control the power of your own happiness. You are who you think you are, and you are as happy as you think you can be.

2. The power to conquer sadness and depression, and achieve happiness, lies inside you. Therapists and medications and external forces can make a difference, but the ultimate power belongs to you, nobody else. You are the master of your emotional destiny.

3. Roughly 50 percent of your happiness is genetic and 10 percent is based on your life circumstances, but you can use simple techniques to boost the whopping 40 percent that lies in your direct control, and thereby achieve significant increases in your emotional well-being.

4. Just as your perceptions of events can trigger downward spirals into depression, you can use positive emotions to ignite magnificent upward spirals of happiness, to heights of emotional thriving and flourishing.

5. The way you treat your body with your diet and exercise can have a sharp positive impact on your happiness.

6. The way you treat your soul with your spiritual journeys can have a sharp positive impact on your happiness.

7. With the proper understanding, tools, and practice in your daily life, you can achieve lasting increases in your happiness.

You and I deserve a life of true happiness and lasting joy.

There are doorways of happiness that lie within your grasp everywhere, every day, every second of your life.

Let's open them up together—right now.

CHAPTER 1

The Brightest and Darkest Places

am having a heart attack.

"Oh, my God," I think, "I'm having a heart attack right in the middle of a casino lobby in Las Vegas."

A heart attack? Is this how it ends?

It all ends here and now, sprawled on the floor of a Las Vegas hotel?

Are you kidding me?

What flashes through my mind is not a beautiful movie of the greatest moments of my life: marrying my wife, Tara; the births of my children; winning TV awards; graduating from the U.S. Naval Academy; having perfect strangers thank me for some charity work I've done.

Instead, as if I'm a jerk, my mind jumps forward to visualize the movie of the next few minutes, of what's going to happen when I hit that floor.

I keel over on the carpet and my soon-to-be widow kneels over me. Pandemonium breaks out; people are running every which way; a mob flocks around us.

"Look, it's Montel Williams!"

"He's dying! Take a picture!"

"Honey, gimme my camera!"

Everybody's whipping out cell phones and cameras; flashbulbs are popping. Someone tears my shirt off and pounds on my chest. The desk clerk runs over with the defibrillator and blasts me with current as I flop around like a rag doll.

I'm splashed on the cover of the *National Enquirer* and I'm the lead story on *Extra!* and *Entertainment Tonight*. The headlines are screaming:

MONTEL'S SHOCKING DEATH PHOTOS!
MOMENT OF DEATH CAUGHT ON TAPE!
FACE OF DEATH IN THE DESERT—EXCLUSIVE VIDEO!

Look, this is how my mind works. I can't help it. That's what goes through my head as I struggle to stay on my feet and start breathing again.

It's one thirty p.m. on July 2, 2008, and I'm scheduled to play in Ante Up for Africa, a charity celebrity poker tournament to raise funds for Darfur. I'm surrounded by my wife, Tara, and our parents.

I've stepped out of the car and into a wave of blast-furnace, 111-degree desert heat that hits me in the head like a sledgehammer.

I thought this would be a short walk inside, but an open-air red-carpet walkway stretches far out before us and it's way too long. It might only be fifty yards, but it seems endless. There's no way I'll make it, I think. I don't know what to do. I'll never make it inside that building.

As someone living with multiple sclerosis, I deal with a number of physical problems. They range from minor irritations to major complications, two of which are pain in the extremities and extreme sensitivity to heat. A hundred and eleven degrees is no picnic for anyone, but when you've got MS it can feel even more unbearable.

I feel a sharp spasm of neuralgic pain in my lower limbs, and it feels like my feet have caught on fire. This is part of my drill with MS, it happens periodically and I'm used to it, but I just cannot describe the magnitude of the pain to you. It feels like I'm walking with flaming torches strapped around my feet.

Out of nowhere, I have trouble breathing.

I struggle inside, walk up a few steps, and then it really hits me. My body suddenly attacks itself, locking up the muscles in my rib cage and cutting off my breathing. It feels like a giant python is wrapped around my chest, squeezing me with relentless force straight into oblivion.

I cannot breathe.

My chest and rib cage are locked in some kind of apocalyptic spasm, and I cannot pull air into my lungs. I try and try, but no air is coming in. On top of which it seems like my heart is hurting, gripping me with a sensation of naked dread and pure horror. Something is cutting off my diaphragm and choking me to death. This has got to be a heart attack.

My wife gently grips my side and helps push me forward as she supports me, preventing me from falling to one side. I feel my body slowing down, as the signals from my brain to my limbs short-circuit and I begin to wobble.

Since being diagnosed with multiple sclerosis in 1999 I've been very public about my condition, but I've tried hard to avoid falling down or collapsing in public, especially in front of cameras. Call it vanity or pride.

Outwardly, I'm not very visibly afflicted by MS. But sometimes what happens when I'm walking is my brain tries to tell my left leg to move forward, but it shoots straight backward instead. I'll wipe out and fall down on the floor. When that happens in public, it can become a big scene and I get really embarrassed. Suddenly, everybody around knows Montel's fallen and they come to the rescue. My mind gets trapped in a frenzy of extreme embarrassment, paranoia, and depression. Now it's about to hit me, on top of this freaking heart attack.

I stagger through the hotel lobby and find a wall to lean on near a little side room. A Good Samaritan notices my distress and races off to get me a pitcher of ice water. I fall onto a couch in the room as Tara's parents and mine guard the door, blocking onlookers from coming in.

I'm about to call out for an ambulance when, slowly, my chest relaxes, the pain eases, and some air sneaks into my lungs. Then I realize, "Damn, this probably isn't a heart attack. *It's that fricking MS hug!*"

An MS hug is when the muscles in your rib cage lock up, triggering pain, choking, or heart attack–like symptoms. Many people with multiple sclerosis experience it, and they often describe it differently. It's happened to me twice before, but nowhere near this severe.

For twenty minutes I sprawl on the couch and cry like a baby with a loaded diaper as I try to cool down and struggle to breathe normally again. My brain and my emotions are shot to hell.

I feel overwhelmingly, cosmically depressed. It's like I'm in a free fall downward into black despair, on the express elevator to Massive Depression. I feel awful about how embarrassed my wife and our parents must be as they realize I can't even manage to walk into a hotel without a huge melodrama erupting.

I'm due in the event green room in a few minutes to get ready to walk down another red carpet into the casino event, this time with crowds and photographers, but right now I feel like crawling under a rock.

Lying there, I feel a tidal wave of dull black depression, so bad I can barely think. It's a familiar feeling; I've had it before.

Every day, in part because of who I am, and in part because of my medical condition and the side effects of my medications, I struggle with emotional pain and with doubts, fears, regrets, and the insidious, self-defeating syndrome of "negative self-talk."

I cry, I get upset, and I get emotional. Sometimes several times a day. I can't help myself.

*　　*　　*

I suffer from a depression that at times has been incredibly severe.

Depression has pushed me to the very abyss, to the point where I've looked over the edge and wondered, "How in the hell could death be any worse than the way I'm feeling right now?"

I've experienced two types of depression in my life.

The first is the kind where I feel an overwhelming sense of sadness or frustration, kind of like being stuck and unable to move forward. I may be angry and not know how to express it, so I'm discouraged and anxious instead. I find help with this kind of depression by talking out my fears and problems with people I love and someone who is a trained listener, like a therapist.

Sometimes I find if I take a small step, like making a list of people and things I'm grateful for, or taking a walk, it will help to lift my mood.

I've also experienced another kind of depression: major depression, like today in Las Vegas. This feeling started right after I was diagnosed with MS.

During that time, I didn't want to get out of bed; I didn't want to go to work. Just putting a smile on my face seemed to take way too much effort. It's virtually impossible to get motivated if you're feeling this way. If it happens to you, my best advice is to seek professional help immediately. Start with your doctor. Get recommendations for a psychologist or a psychiatrist. Sometimes medication is necessary, and guess what: it's okay! If you're a diabetic, you'd take your insulin, right? So don't hesitate to get help. Help is what saved my life, and it can save yours.

I think the reason that MS hug in the casino lobby triggered such despair is that it was a reminder that I'm sick, that I don't have full control over my body, and there's not much I can do to stop the progress of this illness. Sometimes I ponder the futility of fighting this disease I've got. I'm tired of people looking at me and seeing "the guy with MS." MS is not who I am, just as depression is not who I am.

But as I sat on that couch in the casino, a funny thing started happening.

I started trying to think of positive things, to try to flip the paradigm of this moment from a thoroughly crappy experience into something positive, from a depressed moment into something better than that. I tried to visualize the pain in my body stopping.

A voice deep inside my brain said, "Look for the light. Find something positive to focus on. Find a candle to light up the darkness." If you're in a theater that's totally dark and you light a single candle, that one little candle can illuminate the whole room; if you light up more and more candles you can find your way.

I started trying to find that one little sparkle of light, then another, then another.

I realized I've got two good eyes and a brain that works, and I felt grateful.

I looked at my family and I felt the warmth of our relationships: I saw my wife, the very picture of radiance, beauty, and support, and I saw our parents close by, and I felt loved.

I thought of the spiritual reading I've been doing recently, and the tremendous amount of exercise and healthy eating I enjoy, and it all made me feel strong.

I thought of the event that was about to happen, where hundreds of people were coming together to raise $500,000 to help their fellow human beings in trouble on the other side of the planet. I felt like I was doing something decent for others.

I started feeling proud, and filled with hope and energy.

And I started feeling happy.

I spruced myself up, put on a happy face for the photographers, walked down the red carpet onto the casino floor to play in the poker tournament, and promptly got bounced out of the competition.

I played so poorly I barely lasted an hour in the match. But hey, I made it onto the playing field, didn't I?

Hooray for me!

In those moments on the couch in Las Vegas, I experienced the effects of some astonishing feelings that, taken together, provide glimpses of some of the greatest pathways to conquering sadness and depression and achieving human happiness: intentional positive emotions, gratitude, family love and relationships, diet, exercise, and spirituality.

THE MYSTERY OF HAPPINESS

To me, happiness is not a sustained feeling I've enjoyed throughout my whole life. And it has often been punctuated by times of intense sadness, sometimes simultaneously. But when happiness comes, it is so beautiful. One of the mysteries of my life is that my happiest moments have been fully enjoyed only when looking back on them.

My whole life has been a roller coaster of semisimultaneous euphoria and sadness. The day I graduated from the United States Naval Academy in 1980 was by far one of the happiest, greatest moments of my life. To stand before my parents and friends and accept that diploma was a life-transforming achievement, one of the biggest highs I could dream of, to compete, survive, and even thrive in such a tough environment.

However, I was one of the only people in the history of the Naval Academy not to be commissioned as an officer on the same day. My commission was held back because of an eye problem, which I later found out was probably the beginning of my multiple sclerosis.

There I was, graduating from one of the most elite institutions in America, but the navy was telling me, "You're not good enough to do your job. And by the way, your eyes are so bad you can't be a navy pilot, either."

Today, when I think of that day, I am incredibly happy, but at the time it was bittersweet.

A few years later, I almost missed the birth of my first child, Ashley.

I missed most of the pregnancy, as I was at sea on submarine deployments as a navy special duty intelligence officer. Not only did I spend Thanksgiving on a ship six miles off the coast of Grenada as part of the postinvasion operations, but it looked like I was going to miss Ashley's birth, which made me incredibly sad.

By a stroke of luck, I happened to be home in time to be at the hospital for the delivery. Talk about an unbelievably happy moment!

I'll bet every parent can relate to the feeling of pure, unbounded joy I felt on seeing my first child being born. It was like the sky parted, the heavens opened up, and a revelation appeared, a revelation of the fact that my mortality isn't as important, because now I have a legacy that will live beyond me. And I saw before me the most beautiful child on the planet.

But then a few weeks later, I was back at sea.

I was unable to hold my baby girl in my arms, or hear her cry, or tuck her in to sleep. It was a very tough marriage, in part because I simply wasn't there much of the time. It was a lot like what so many American servicemen and servicewomen deployed to Iraq and Afghanistan are experiencing today: they get married because they're getting shipped overseas three days later. That's it for the next 180 days. They're gone. Then they're home for a week and a half, then gone for another 180 days. It's the toughest thing on a marriage you can imagine.

Professionally, I was immensely happy in my military life. Why? Because the U.S. military is a society within a society where everyone has to both believe and live the basic tenets that all men are created equal, with justice for all.

I also had very happy moments in 1989 and 1990 when I came off active duty, started my own company, and saw my career as a speaker go through the roof. I was a young man who caught the eye of the nation: I was a finalist for *Time* magazine's Man of the Year, I spoke at

Fortune magazine's education summit, and I was even asked to speak at the White House. Then at lightning speed, I successfully negotiated a deal for my own TV talk show without an agent or a manager.

Unfortunately, at the same time, I was meeting with lawyers to finalize the paperwork for a divorce.

Last year, my book *Living Well* was rocketing onto three bestseller lists—the *New York Times*, the *Wall Street Journal*, and *Publishers Weekly*—at the same time the clock was ticking down to my last taping of my talk show, which had been canceled after seventeen years on the air.

I have these huge highs at the same time I'm riding the terrible lows. Maybe that's happened to you, too; maybe that's a natural course of life.

And then there are those days when your whole life changes with a single phone call.

THE DAY I GOT FIRED

"Montel, it's over. It's just over."

The voice on the phone sounded like the bark of an elderly bulldog filtered through a sack of gravel.

The voice belonged to one of my TV bosses.

He was a giant in the business, a legendary salesman and deal maker.

And he was firing me.

Just a few weeks later, he would drop dead from a stroke. He was only in his early sixties, the likely victim of decades of endless business travel, mountains of hotel food, and oceans of booze.

Let's just call him Fred, which isn't his real name. I think the dead are entitled to a certain degree of respect.

He launched the careers of people like Oprah, Dr. Phil, and Rachael Ray. A few years back he had cashed in a cool few billion dollars for himself in a mega–business deal and he became absorbed into the corporate structure.

But he seemed to me to be in bad health for a long time, and it always looked to me like he could keel over any minute from obesity and lack of fresh air. His gargantuan drinking binges were the stuff of many unprintable stories in the TV business. I'm not judging him for his problem with alcohol. He was very open about it, and he'd licked the bottle years before. But it looked to me like it had already had a terrible impact on him.

Right now I was speechless and experiencing something like an out-of-body experience. I could almost feel myself being lifted up by forces I couldn't control and thrown down on a different track of life, the destination of which I couldn't see.

Most of us get fired at some point in our lives. It can be a routine bump on the road of life: you pick yourself up, shake it off, and start all over again. Or you can free-fall into massive depression and catastrophic feelings of despair.

Me? I'd never been fired before in my life, so at first I had no idea how to feel.

I was completing my seventeenth year on the air with my talk show. I was already thinking that maybe this was long enough to stay in one gig; maybe it was time to launch something new. I was thinking about what I could do next, and how I could get out of my existing contract. But I figured we were good for maybe one or two more seasons on the air.

By most measures, we were enjoying a tremendously successful run. I'd been on the air for almost an entire generation, we'd produced thirty-two hundred shows, had over twenty-two thousand guests on the program, and I'd won practically every award in the TV business. And after years of fierce competition we were surviving and thriving among key audiences. Day after day we were still tackling tough issues, and helping people live their lives better. Four million people were watching me every day.

Personally and professionally, I was flourishing. A few weeks earlier I'd married Tara at a beautiful ceremony with family and friends on the beach in Bermuda. I was working out every day, eating very healthy, and enjoying some fascinating and rewarding spiritual journeys. I had just put the finishing touches on my last book, *Living Well*, which soon blasted off the bookstore shelves and became an instant national best-seller.

I had called Fred to talk about some good news: the ratings of the *Montel Williams Show*. In the normal life cycle of most TV shows, especially those on the air as long as mine, you're going to take some hard hits in the ratings, and ratings will erode over time. Mine was no exception. But today I had good news for Fred: our ratings were popping this season.

Fred came on the line. "I want to let you know we're having a great November sweeps," I told him. "Ratings are looking good. They're going up all season!"

"Yeah, yeah," said Fred, "but you're not doing well on Fox stations."

Right away, this struck me as weird. The tone of his voice told me something was way, way off here.

I countered, "But across the board we're doing great."

He let off a long, awful wheezing cough, and finally said, "You know what? I guess I might as well tell you now. You're done. You're just done."

"What do you mean, I'm done?" I asked.

"Well, we're not picking up your show."

"*What?*" It felt like he'd dropped a bomb on my head. I had no warning this was coming.

"Montel, it's over. It's just over. You had a good run, Montel," said Fred. "Just be happy you had a good run."

I had just gotten off the phone with the other TV executives who oversaw my show, none of whom had an inkling this was in the works. Fred was part of a corporate structure, but he was so powerful that he could act as independently and arbitrarily as he pleased.

It turns out that Fred had been wheeling and dealing behind my back to undermine and kill off my show and replace it with a project he thought could make more money for him. He was doing this behind everybody's back for six or seven months, keeping it secret even from people in his own company. That's how Hollywood works sometimes. They'll stab you in the throat or in the ass, all in a day's work.

This felt like a really ugly way to get fired.

I hung up the phone, turned to Melanie McLaughlin, who has managed my companies for nineteen years, and said, "We just got freaking fired."

She said, *"What?"*

I could have fallen apart. I could have jumped out the window. I could have let it ruin my holiday season. It could have been the most depressed and anxiety-ridden period of my whole life.

I could have been angry as hell. I could have let it completely derail me and I could have given up hope.

But I didn't. Instead I felt energized and liberated.

And yes, in a strange way I felt really happy.

"Okay," I said to no one in particular, "what's next?"

One tough thing was that for business reasons I had to keep this a secret for the next few months until it was formally announced by the company. I played along, to be nice to the company that fired me. I had to bounce around the country like a happy idiot, holding the ugly truth inside me.

But overall, it was a really positive turning point in my life. The timing decision had been taken from me, but I had already stepped onto this path; this just got me moving faster. Today I've got three new TV shows in development, I am creating a new global poker league, I'm

CEO of a company developing diet and health-related products and equipment, and tomorrow I'm addressing the Baltimore City Council about a low-to-medium-income housing project I'm developing. Maybe I have some kind of Business Attention Deficit Disorder!

So I got fired. And I came through it a wiser and better person.

Isn't it strange, though, how sometimes the *little* things in life can knock you off track emotionally?

Take what happened to me last month, for example.

I was at JFK Airport, scheduled to get on a six a.m. business flight.

Because of my digestive problems connected to multiple sclerosis, I can't eat most airline food anymore, so I take a green vegetable–and-fruit smoothie in a plastic bottle with me whenever I fly. It's delicious and superhealthy. I carry a doctor's note with me to get it through security, written exactly as the Transportation Safety Authority instructed me. It usually works fine and I get right through security, no sweat. I've done this two or three hundred times.

Not today. I put the letter and the bottle through the X-ray machine after explaining it to a nice TSA employee.

Then I stepped through the metal detector and was greeted by another TSA officer, but this guy looked like he wanted to declare war on me. For whatever reason, he decided he was going to put me through the mill.

He grabbed the bottle and declared, "You can't have this."

I said, "Yes, Officer, but I have this note from a doctor, written the way the TSA requires."

"Don't tell me my job!" he shouted. "I have to test it!"

He opened up the bottle, put his dirty-gloved fingers inside, poked around and poured a sample out to be tested for explosives. In other words, he totally fouled up the contents, rendering it undrinkable. Hey, would you drink a smoothie after I'd scraped my mitts around it with a nasty rubber glove?

It was only five o'clock in the morning and I was already hurting physically and emotionally, and this fellow was yelling at me in front of a small crowd of people.

He gave me the bottle back. I felt he'd been way out of line, so I said, "Let me speak to a supervisor, please."

"I am a supervisor!" he exclaimed. *"And I will throw your ass out of here, right now!"*

By now I was shaking with anger and anxiety, and my heart was banging in my chest. Even worse, I was hungry, but this character had basically taken my food away, so I'd be starving all through the flight and into the afternoon. I was ready to scream.

I walked away from the desk over to my gate and sat there weeping for literally twenty minutes. I should not have let this guy get to me, but he hit me at the wrong time.

I wanted to complain to someone, so I got security over from Delta Airlines. They called the person in charge of security at the airport to come over and console me. Bottom line: nothing got done.

When I read about things like this happening to celebrities, I usually laugh and think, "Get over yourself, for God's sake, you idiot!" That's right: grow up, Montel! Don't be such a baby! Thank the TSA for protecting you so well when you travel!

But that stupid little incident left me shaking, a quivering helpless pile of human wreckage, and it bothered me emotionally for weeks. I would think back on it and start crying. I couldn't let it go.

I think it was because, like that day in Las Vegas, it was a dramatic reminder that I am sick.

I'm sick of being sick. Being sick sucks! I take forty pills and three shots a day. My whole day is an intricate process of little physical maneuvers, kind of a symphony, to avoid falling down, to move forward without crutches or a wheelchair. I keep telling myself I'm not sick. And it felt like the TSA guy slapped me in the face and said, "Hey, dummy, remember this—you're sick!"

THIS IS MONTEL ON DRUGS

I stick a needle in my leg three times a day and shoot it with a drug.

One of the shots is a very promising drug for the management of MS that is believed to help modulate the immune system. I believe it is literally helping to keep me alive on this planet. It's one of an exciting whole new generation of medications designed to help people with MS live better lives. Lots of people take this particular drug with no problems at all.

But some people do experience side effects, including mood swings. These hit me in really strange ways. For example, yesterday I was on an airplane and I watched a movie in which the father character dies. This made me cry loudly and uncontrollably in my airplane seat. I started feeling really stupid for crying in public, and then I was really off to the races! This quickly led to my feeling like a total failure, which made me cry even more. I eventually bounced out of it, but it was such a strange feeling.

Until I started taking this MS drug a few years ago, and before I was diagnosed with MS, I would never have described myself as having major depression.

Thinking back on it, I realize now that the intensely emotional subject matter of my shows didn't help. If you take a person like me who can get depressed, and give him a job dealing with emotional turmoil every day, what you've got is a recipe for a train wreck. After taping TV shows dealing with everybody else's problems all week, on top of the drug, on top of trying to manage the symptoms of MS, by Friday mornings I'd be a wreck. I'd spend an hour or two in the bathroom crying, to try to expel the tumult going on in my head.

You know what the number-one cause of death is among people with multiple sclerosis? It's suicide. I think it's from the physical disabilities and depression brought on by the disease and by chemical imbalances in the brain, perhaps sometimes on top of all the medicine we have to take.

Before I got MS, when doctors would ask me, "Have you ever suffered from mood problems?" I'd say, "Hell, no!" Sure, I had periods of sadness, anger, and anxiety, and I've always been a passionate guy, and pretty open about my feelings. When I was in the military, I was extremely intense and sometimes emotionally angry in my desire to succeed. I was trained and ready to slit the throat of the enemy. But depressed? No way! It was a foreign concept to me. MS changed all that.

I started getting depressed. I took the depression grand tour: light depression, moderate depression, and kick-ass severe depression. Then doctors started prescribing me different drugs for depression and the real fun began.

I am a 100 percent supporter of Western medicine, with all its miracles and its imperfections. I'm also wide-open to critical opinions and alternative approaches. In my opinion, when the pharmaceutical companies do something we disagree with, we should tell them. And when they create a drug that helps us live a better life, or saves lives, we should cheer them on. I work with leading pharmaceutical and research companies and their trade association PhRMA, as spokesperson for the Partnership for Prescription Assistance, a fantastic program that is the proudest professional achievement in my life so far.

Some antidepression drugs are absolute lifesavers for many patients. But drugs are not always perfect for different patients, and obviously neither are doctors. I'm living proof. For my bouts of depression, I was prescribed a broad spectrum of drugs over time, from mild antipsychotics all the way to antiseizure medications.

When I was on an antiseizure medication, I felt like a zombie. It made me feel cloudy and disconnected from everything. When I spoke, the words sounded like a jumble of mass confusion. I could feel my creative edge and mental sharpness blunt and fade, and I hated the feeling.

Then I was put on an antidepressant medicine. I won't name it, because my experience may not be typical. I can tell you it wasn't Prozac. This drug made me feel agitated, psychotic, and eventually suicidal. I was having serious conversations in my brain about how to kill myself. Should I jump out the window? Jump in front of traffic? Suck a bullet out of a gun barrel? I'm a gun owner, so this is an extra-dangerous thought process for me.

After a personal problem one day, I found myself standing in the doorway of my office and I heard myself announcing to my staff, "You know what? Maybe I should just blow my brains out!" This freaked me out so badly that I immediately grabbed my prescription bottle and flushed the pills down the toilet. (I later found out from a doctor that this is a bad idea. Rather than stop cold turkey, he said, I should have weaned myself off the drug under medical supervision.)

Right now, I'm not taking any medication. Some doctors might look at me and say I'm a perfect candidate for this drug or that drug, but I feel okay without them right now. Some people are opposed to any antidepressant medicine at all. That's their personal choice. But I'll tell you: I'm convinced that medications help some people function better, deal with depression, and enjoy life more.

I NEED PROFESSIONAL HELP

Those four words can be the most important words of your life.

The World Health Organization defines depression this way: "Depression is a common mental disorder that presents with depressed mood, loss of interest or pleasure, feelings of guilt or low self-worth, disturbed sleep or appetite, low energy, and poor concentration. These problems can become chronic or recurrent and lead to substantial impairments in an individual's ability to take care of his or her everyday responsibilities."

If you feel you might be depressed, you really should seek out professional help and see what treatment and therapy options are available. Don't feel ashamed, or bashful, or afraid. Depression can truly be a silent killer. I strongly believe that if you even think you're depressed, then you need to see a doctor. Don't wait. Do it now. You'll be amazed how much the right doctor and the right information can help you. Trust me, I know it.

I've been in psychiatric therapy several times in my life.

You should be simultaneously very open-minded and ruthlessly skeptical in evaluating therapy.

What do I mean by ruthlessly skeptical? I mean you should always keep in mind that doctors are fallible, they need your help to get things right, and they are there to serve you, not the other way around. You are the boss of your own medical care, and it's your job to lead the process, gather information, and question everything.

I have had great therapists who have helped me navigate personal crises and helped me lift myself up and live a much happier life. They have become very positive figures in my life.

And I have had a lousy therapist or two who have pushed me down emotionally and frankly made things worse, so bad that I didn't want any more therapy. So I did the same thing you should do if it happens to you—I fired them.

One psychologist I saw was an incredibly gloomy, maudlin character who acted like he was sorry you had to see him. When I first met him he looked at me like he was Sigmund Freud reviewing the case of a hopelessly deranged person. Other times, his expression matched that of a doctor who's about to tell you you've got something terminal. I'd walk out of his office feeling more depressed than when I went in!

In the middle of a therapy session, another psychiatrist suddenly became inflamed over something I said, and he started screaming at me. Then he got a grip on himself, apologized, and gave me a soliloquy about how I had triggered the memory of something his father had said to him when he was a kid. Some psychiatrists are pretty screwed up themselves!

But the good psychotherapists I've seen have helped me live a better emotional life. They've helped me work through personal crises, validated the good things in my life, and helped me help myself. They've understood that their job isn't to direct my behavior, but to help me explore my own emotional problems and solutions. They've been a tremendous help to me in my journey toward happiness.

While researching this book, I interviewed one of the top psychiatrists in New York, Dr. Richard Rosenthal of St. Luke's Roosevelt Hospital Center. He has an enormous track record of clinical experience treating thousands of patients. I'd never met him before. He bounded out of his office to greet me with a huge smile on his face and he seemed to crackle with positive energy.

As we sat down to talk, I was struck by how open, enthusiastic, and nonjudgmental he was about his work, and about my emotions and my ideas. It struck me that a big reason he was so successful in his work is that he comes across like a powerfully positive life coach, someone who would really be your champion. "The next time I feel the need to formally consult a psychiatrist," I thought, "this is exactly the kind of doctor I'd want to talk to." I think that's the kind of doctor you should try to find if you need one.

The journey toward happiness can be helped tremendously by skilled guides like a good therapist, a loving and wise parent, a member of the clergy, or a good friend. But I believe the voyage starts deep inside yourself.

It's funny, but for me, writing this book is like good therapy.

It's making me happy by helping me better recognize, and understand, and savor the moments of happiness in my life. It really is a glorified personal journal. It's like a therapeutic exercise.

And it's helping me understand that maybe it's okay for me to be many things emotionally. Maybe it's okay for me to be sometimes sad, sometimes depressed, and other times very happy. Maybe it's okay for me to be all of the above more or less simultaneously.

You know what?

Maybe I'm just human!

How can you and I discover the keys to live well emotionally and start building a life of happiness?

A wonderful place to start is deep within our own minds, where we can explore the ancient question of what happiness is, and what it really means.

CHAPTER 2

A Journey of the Mind

Happiness is the Holy Grail of Life.

It has been a human obsession as far back as Aristotle, who declared happiness "the meaning and the purpose of life, the whole aim and end of human existence." In the twentieth century the Dalai Lama agreed: "I believe that the very purpose of our life is to seek happiness. That is clear, whether one believes in religion or not, whether one believes in this religion or that religion. We all are seeking something better in life. So I think the very motion of our life is toward happiness." The American founding fathers went so far as to enshrine "the pursuit of happiness" in the Declaration of Independence as an inalienable right of mankind.

But what exactly is happiness?

What does it mean? What is it supposed to feel like?

There are almost 6.8 billion people on Earth right now, and there are probably that many answers to those questions.

Happiness is, in fact, an elusive, nebulous creature of swirling paradoxes.

It is everywhere, but it can be maddeningly difficult to grasp.

When you have it, you may not fully realize it at the time.

We think we know what it is, but we have real trouble putting it into words.

On my TV show one day, I sent cameras out and asked people, "What does happiness mean to you?" Everybody had a different opinion.

One man offered a Zen-like thought: "You cannot own happiness. You cannot touch happiness. You only can feel happiness."

"Happiness is contagious!" laughed one woman.

"I'm happy right now, very happy," said another. Why? "I'm in the shopping mall!"

A young man on the street pondered the question and replied, "Sky-diving. I really want to go skydiving. That would make my life right there."

One couple agreed on the essence of their happiness. "A lot of food," said the guy. "We eat a lot of food!" His female companion chimed right in, "Yeah, food—food makes us happy!"

"I love money. I love food. I love jewelry. I love clothes. I love all those kinds of material things," declared another woman.

"I'm not a materialistic person," countered one man, "I just like family and friends." Other responses:

"When you see somebody and you smile at them, and they smile at you back."

"If I didn't have to work, I would be a lot happier."

"Being happy—I believe it's the beginning of being healthy."

"I think they actually say happiness and laughter add eight years to your life."

"Yeah! Laughter is the best kind of medicine."

"What would make my mother happy is for me to find a nice woman to marry one day."

"Now I'm divorced. That's why I'm happy!"

"Getting my braces taken off would make me really, really happy."

Happiness is a common denominator across all mankind, but it is frustratingly hard to define. Dictionaries are fuzzy, offering platitudes like "a state of well-being and contentment," "a pleasurable or satisfying experience," or "good fortune." Philosophers aren't much more help. "What is happiness?" asked Friedrich Nietzsche. "The feeling that power increases, that resistance is overcome." Henry Wadsworth Longfellow said simply, "To be strong is to be happy." Well, okay, if you say so.

When President John F. Kennedy was asked by a reporter about happiness, he quoted the ancient Greek definition that happiness is "full use of your powers along lines of excellence."

One way of thinking about happiness is to see it endure in the face of terrible adversity and overwhelming odds.

I once had an extraordinary young man named Harold Dennis on my TV show. He was in the worst drunk-driving accident in American history. He was burned on 40 percent of his body, including third-degree burns on his face, neck, and shoulders.

Harold recalled the moment of impact when a drunken driver in a pickup truck drove straight into his school bus and detonated the gas tank:

> My sister and I went on a local church outing to King's Island Amusement Park up in Cincinnati, Ohio. It was an exciting day running around with your friends.
>
> Little did we know that our lives were going to change forever that night.
>
> Approximately ten fifty-five that evening, we were coming southbound on Interstate 71 and a truck hit the bus. The impact jarred me into the seat in front of me. I remember hearing everyone screaming and tires screeching and the bus came to a stop.
>
> It was at that instant when the bus exploded.
>
> At that point it was mass chaos. Raging fire, pitch-black dark, the

odds were stacked against everyone in there. We had sixty-three people on this one bus. It was a death trap.

At the rear exit, I was met with bodies piled from the floor to the ceiling. Everybody was trying to get out. I just kind of tried to weasel my way through and I fell out along with about four or five other people.

I spent about the next two months of my life recovering. I spent a few weeks in the intensive-care unit not knowing if I was going to make it.

It was quite a while before I was able to see my face in a mirror for the first time.

I didn't recognize the person looking back at me.

Harold spent ten weeks in the hospital, had more than a dozen skin grafts along with treatments for severe lung damage and emotional trauma. He was only fourteen years old. Twenty-four children and three adults were killed in the disaster and many of the thirty-six survivors were injured.

Harold Dennis's dream of happiness was just to have a normal life and maybe have a nice girl fall in love with him someday. "I knew that I would find happiness eventually," he remembered. "Happiness for me was being able to interact and walk the streets proudly and be able to live my life like others."

AMERICA'S GREAT EMOTIONAL DEPRESSION

America has always been consumed with the quest for happiness, but in many ways, America today seems to be an extremely unhappy country.

In fact, I believe America is in the midst of a largely undiagnosed national depression, the magnitude of which we have not felt since the Great Depression itself.

We are experiencing an epidemic of anxiety, sadness, and emotional turmoil.

Our emotional health as a nation is a disaster in progress.

We are in the midst of a Great Emotional Depression.

I have an unusual theory about our national depression. It started in the 1960s and 1970s with assassinations, Vietnam, and Watergate, but I think it was exacerbated sharply in 1998 with the Monica Lewinsky scandal. We were overwhelmed with sordid details about our national father figure, the president, cheating on his wife and lying about it to sabotage a sexual harassment lawsuit, leading to his impeachment in the House of Representatives.

We should have undergone some kind of national psychotherapy for this traumatic national family event. But it was too gross, too embarrassing. America simply did not discuss its family drama in a meaningful psychological way. We quickly recoiled and ran away from it as soon as we could. I think this added to our dysfunction as a society and as a national family.

In the decade since then we have endured an election debacle, the horrors of 9/11 and Hurricane Katrina, and bloody wars in Iraq and Afghanistan that have seen thousands of Americans killed, and hundreds of thousands come home physically and mentally wounded.

It's like we are wired into a steady intravenous flow of bad news.

We have watched twenty-four-hour coverage of earthquakes, tsunamis, floods, terrorism, pestilence, school massacres, obesity crises, road rage, air rage, domestic violence, and family members killing each other. During one week in 2008, some two hundred thousand souls in China and Burma left our planet at almost the same time. The real estate market plunged, hundreds of thousands of home owners faced foreclosure, and Wall Street imploded, as food and gas prices shot up, perhaps never to come back down.

Sometimes it feels like we're living in some kind of national psychosis. It seems every other day there's a bomb threat in American schools, or a child kidnapped, or a clergy sex abuse scandal.

> ᏮᏮ *We are in the midst of an epidemic of depression, one*
> *with consequences that, through suicide, takes as many*
> *lives as the AIDS epidemic and is more widespread.*
>
> —Dr. Martin Seligman, University of Pennsylvania
> Psychiatry Professor

One of the major triggers of depression is the sense that we're overwhelmed with problems to which there are no solutions—and the media barrages us every day with seemingly hopeless problems. All these external things can affect us on a personal level, and affect our mood every single day.

At the same time, we live in a paradoxical state of avoidance and outright denial over the immensity of the human tragedy and mental health crisis that's brewing in the minds of our soldiers coming home from war.

We've sent a million men and women in and out of Iraq and Afghanistan. Many of those brave souls who have been hurt physically or emotionally are coming home with profound mental health issues and challenges that we are all going to have to grapple with together, as a national family, for decades to come.

It's not like it used to be, when many Vietnam veterans were out of sight and out of mind, in long-term rehab or living in homeless shelters or cardboard boxes. The miracles of modern battlefield medicine have enabled so many soldiers to survive getting arms, legs, and eyes blown off, and now they're back home, stepping up to civilian life. These veterans are coming back and rightly demanding to be contributing members of society, to get their jobs back, to make a difference.

In early 2008 I caused a big controversy when I appeared on the TV show *Fox and Friends*.

I was invited on the show to talk about my health-and-fitness book *Living Well*.

But when I got to the green room to get ready to go on air, I was told the three hosts wanted to talk instead about a Hollywood star who had just died from a drug overdose. I said there was no way I want to talk about that. Not only was his body barely cold, but I did not know him. The media was in a frenzied orgy of coverage of the man's death, and frankly it disgusted me.

On the air, I kept my cool and stayed respectful, but I got really pissed about what happened next.

The clip, titled "Fox Turns the Tables on a Fox Morning Television Show," was posted on YouTube. So far, it's been viewed over 830,000 times. Here's what happened:

Fox Host: An actor gone way too soon. The tragedy: a major one. Was the pressure of stardom too much for the young actor? Someone who knows how it can be under the glare of the celebrity microscope is Montel Williams, who joins us in the studio this morning.

Montel: Good morning. Thanks for having me.

Host: It's good to have you here. Boy, we talk about a tragic situation: Heath Ledger. Weigh in on that for us.

Montel: You know, for me, I've gotta tell you, my heart goes out to his family. But I have been repulsed, honestly, by all the coverage. Here's a question I have: watch this. How many people have died in Iraq since January first?

Host: It's about . . . it's about twenty.

Montel: No. It's not about. It is twenty-eight.

Host: Okay, look, excuse me, Montel—

Montel: I say it that way because we're gonna spend fifteen minutes talking about this. I've not seen one death, one name of a soldier, one person who allows us to do this, and you were in the military. We're the ones who defend this democracy. Those guys are over there dying, and we're gonna sit here and speculate about a young man who passed away, who's somebody's child, who's somebody's father, has not even been buried yet, and I think it's gone way too far.

Host: But why do we do that as a society? I mean—

Montel: Because it is this voracious appetite to bring on ratings. That's what it is. We know it. We know it as a fact. Let's be honest about it.

Host: Of course it's ratings, but it's the appetite—we're feeding the beast. The audience is tuning in to that.

Montel: Yeah, well, cart before the horse—horse before the cart—I don't know who drives it. I think if right now we woke up this morning and instead of talking about Heath Ledger we talked about the trooper who died last night by the IED—

Host: Montel, Montel, we have numbers. I mean, look, I . . . I . . . I . . . It's kind of a sad reality, though. I mean, troops have been dying in Iraq since March of 2003, correct?

Montel: And we don't talk about them.

Host: Well, I mean, look, we talk about the war plenty. I was actually embedded. I was there for the invasion. I mean . . . we . . . I think everybody in this country knows we're at war.

Montel: Nobody in this country knows who died yesterday. And if I know about Heath, I wanna know about the troops. That's it.

Host: We talk about Heath because he was an icon. He was someone that really stood out.

Montel: And I admire him. My heart goes out to him. I didn't know him. And there are a lot of people. Yesterday, probably in this country, another four hundred people passed away. I don't know any of them.

Host: Is there any realistic way to talk about four hundred people who died individually?

Montel: All of the troops yesterday, and I'm sorry, let's have this discussion about Heath Ledger, but I want to tell America: twenty-eight troops died since January first. That's what I want to talk about, for me. Now, I mean, you guys can do it if you want. It's cool. I'm not gonna knock you. Talk about it if that's part of what you do, and that's part of what we need for ratings. I don't need them.

They soon broke for a commercial, saying I'd be back for the next segment to discuss my new book, *Living Well*. Well, I didn't come back. Based on what happened, I decided to say good-bye and walk out of that building.

That exchange illustrated the kind of avoidance and denial that feeds our national emotional depression and collective dysfunction, and I believe in the long run prevents us from pursuing happiness in a meaningful, healthy way.

I think our Great National Depression helps to explain how Barack Obama and Sarah Palin exploded into the American consciousness. Both Obama and Palin were breaths of brand-new political air that came from way out of left and right field and set much of the country on fire. After years of dreary, ossified political discourse, they connected powerfully with Americans who were yearning for hope, for youth, for inspiration, for new ideas, and yes, for *change*.

Look at the images and stereotypes Barack Obama shattered. Ever since this nation began, the image of black men has often been of an oppressed, threatening, angry, uneducated underclass condemned to perpetual despair and defeat, as victims unworthy and even incapable of any true happiness. In my lifetime, black Americans in the Deep South were being stripped of every vestige of human and political rights and treated as subhuman. Even today, black men have terribly high unemployment rates, and nearly half of young American black men have spent time in the criminal justice system.

Suddenly, in 2008, the idea of electing a young black man as president of the United States became a flesh-and-blood reality. It is an idea so revolutionary to America and the world that we haven't absorbed it yet. It is huge. It is spectacular. It is history-changing and it is psyche-changing. I think it will transform our national emotional well-being in ways we don't yet understand.

But right now, as a nation, we are so apparently unhappy that over 100 million prescriptions for antidepressants are written every year, and the treatment of children and adolescents with antianxiety medication is becoming routine. A lot of people in this country are hurting. Many of them are hurting and don't even know why, and may be too afraid or ashamed to seek the help they desperately need.

By one estimate, over 80 percent of depressed patients could benefit from treatment, yet almost two-thirds won't get help, as they may feel too paralyzed or stigmatized by their condition.

Consider these stark statistics:

- Depression affects almost 10 percent of the U.S. adult population each year.
- About 17 percent of the U.S. population will suffer from a major depressive episode at some point in their lifetime.
- Up to half of female adolescents, and half of the elderly, may be affected by depression.
- Depression is one of the leading causes of disability in America, costing the nation over $40 billion annually in lost work and medical expenses.
- Data in recent decades suggests a virtual explosion in the reported cases of depression, a 300 percent increase in the decade ending in 1997, for example, which probably results in part from greater awareness and improved diagnosis.
- The number of people using SSRIs like Prozac and other newer antidepressants almost doubled from 1996 to 2001. Their use among children, adolescents, and the elderly increased by between 200 percent and 300 percent during the 1990s.
- From 1996 to 2001, total spending on antidepressants jumped from $3.4 billion to $7.9 billion.
- By the year 2000, antidepressants were the top-selling group of drugs in America.
- The World Health Organization considers depression the leading cause of disability for women of all ages. The WHO projects that by 2020, depression will rank as the number-two cause of global disability after heart disease.

In the face of these odds, should we even try to attain such an elusive thing as happiness? Is it an object of desire as distant and impossible to obtain as the mythical Holy Grail?

THE VALUE OF SADNESS

Wait a second.

Even if we could achieve a life of happiness, why should we even want to be happy all the time?

Some people argue that you shouldn't even bother to go looking for happiness. Forget it, they say, it's a self-canceling idea. A Japanese proverb describes the pursuit of happiness as "clutching a shadow or chasing the wind."

In Rome in the first century BC, a performance artist named Publilius Syrus declared, "To call yourself happy is to provoke disaster." Albert Einstein dismissed the quest for happiness as complete nonsense. "Well-being and happiness never appeared to me as an absolute aim," he declared. "I am even inclined to compare such moral aims to the ambitions of a pig. The ideals that have lighted my way are Kindness, Beauty, and Truth." The British philosopher John Stuart Mill argued: "Ask yourself whether you are happy and you cease to be so."

And what's wrong with sadness? "Is life satisfaction always great?" asked the great investor John Templeton. "Maybe a little bit of dissatisfaction is okay."

After all, some of our greatest minds have done some of their best work while in the throes of melancholy, sadness, or flat-out depression: Winston Churchill, Abraham Lincoln, Beethoven, and Vincent van Gogh, to name a few. The great French playwright Moliere announced that "unbroken happiness is a bore; one should have ups and downs in life." George Bernard Shaw agreed, arguing that a lifetime of happiness would be "hell on earth."

Aren't personal crises, loss, sadness, and periods of emotional darkness just part of human nature? Absolutely! They can help us grow, and become stronger, and change ourselves for the better. Ed Diener, a professor of psychology at the University of Illinois, has argued that when you're in a negative mood, "you become more analytical, more critical and more innovative. You need negative emotions, including sadness, to direct your thinking." Critical thinking, fear, and skepticism can all be healthy and normal, and critical to our survival in the face of danger and uncertainty.

Professor Diener has a fascinating theory about the dangers of too much happiness. In the scientific journal *Perspectives on Psychological Science*, he and his colleagues wrote that based on their research, "once a moderate level of happiness is achieved, further increases can sometimes be detrimental" to success, earning power, and education. On a "happiness scale" of 1 to 10, with 10 meaning extremely happy, the "8s" earned more and were better educated than the "10s." It could be that the people who have some discontent in their lives are more motivated to improve themselves. "If you're totally satisfied with your life and with how things are going in the world," said Diener, "you don't feel very motivated to work for change. Be wary when people tell you you should be happier."

Negative experiences can lead to change, and therefore eventually to happiness. As a Chinese proverb explains, "Without scaling mountains no one can know the height of heaven; without descending valleys, no one can know the depth of the earth." As the Dalai Lama put it, "The person who has had more experience of hardships can stand more firmly in the face of problems than the person who has never experienced suffering."

⟡ *Suffering produces endurance,*
and endurance produces character,
and character produces hope.

—Paul, Letter to the Romans

The times when you have great turmoil in your life can turn out to be exactly the moments that trigger positive turning points and open you up to new horizons of potential. The author Radmilla Moacanin wrote of these times, "These are borderline states; they are times of crisis, when the tension is at its peak, but which are also most pregnant psychologically, since they are times when change can most readily occur. Inherent in such states is the opportunity for transformation. In the crack between two worlds—of the living and the dead, of death and rebirth—lies the supreme opportunity."

There has been a happiness craze in America, with scores of books and TV shows devoted to allegedly quick and easy ways to get happy. But as the Harvard psychology professor Tal Ben-Shahar has said, "There are no shortcuts. There is no 'happiness now,' no 'five easy steps to happiness.'"

Happiness is actually part of the often-hard work of life, and it involves integrating periods of sadness into our lives. When you think about it, without sadness the idea of happiness has little meaning. "Sadness is inevitable," said Professor Ben-Shahar. "A full and fulfilling life is not a life that is devoid of painful emotions. There are only two kinds of people who don't experience painful emotions: the psychopath and dead people."

And in an incredible intellectual twist, two experts are arguing that it turns out we may not be as depressed as we thought we were, and that *up to 25 percent of those who qualify for diagnosis of major depressive disorder under current criteria may not really have the condition.* There is, they believe, a massive design flaw in the way depression psychiatry is currently constructed.

> ≋ *Sadness is an inherent part of the human condition, not a mental disorder.*
>
> —Professors Jerome Wakefield and Allan Horwitz

The two experts are Allan Horwitz, dean of social and behavioral sciences at Rutgers University, and Jerome C. Wakefield, professor of social work and psychiatry and a mental health researcher at New York University. In their groundbreaking 2007 book *The Loss of Sadness*, they argue that there is a critical difference between intense sadness, a normal, natural human emotion, and depression, which is a mental disorder requiring treatment. I bet most experts would agree with that.

But here's the point with which they attempt to shake the pillars of psychology: they argue very strongly that the current definition of major depressive disorder, as set forth in the technical bible of the psychiatric profession, the *DSM* (which stands for *Diagnostic and Statistical Manual of Mental Disorders*), is way too broad and results in many cases of normal sadness being misdiagnosed as clinical depression.

As an exercise, let's see how you stack up against this widely used definition of depression.

Could You Fit the Definition of Depressed?
Depression Checklist

Check off which, if any, of these symptoms you have experienced for the last two weeks:

___ Depressed mood.

___ Diminished interest or pleasure in activities.

___ Weight gain or loss or change in appetite.

___ Insomnia or hypersomnia (excessive sleep).

___ Psychomotor agitation (speeding up) or retardation (slowing down).

___ Fatigue or loss of energy.

____ Feelings of worthlessness or excessive or inappropriate guilt.

____ Diminished ability to think or concentrate or indecisiveness.

____ Recurrent thoughts of death or suicidal ideation or suicide attempt.

If you checked off five of the above symptoms as happening to you through the period of the last two weeks, and two of the five include #1 and #2, the *DSM* says you fit the diagnosis of major depressive disorder.

If this is the case, I believe that to be safe you should contact a mental health professional for a full evaluation. The *DSM* does say that patients are exempt from diagnosis if their symptoms are due to "a normal period of bereavement after the death of a loved one," which lasts no more than two months and does not include most severe symptoms, like thinking about suicide.

But here's a catch. Professors Wakefield and Horwitz argue that some people could experience five of the above symptoms for two weeks, including #1 and #2, just by feeling sad, not depressed. They could feel that way after any number of very stressful life events, like losing a job, betrayal by a romantic partner, not being promoted, flunking a big test, or getting diagnosed with a major illness. Having the symptoms in these contexts could be a normal human reaction of intense sadness, Wakefield and Horwitz assert, not a disorder or genuine psychiatric disturbance.

Due to what they call this "semantic confusion" of normal sadness and depressive mental disorder, Wakefield and Horwitz conclude that up to 25 percent of depression diagnoses may be "false positives," or wrong. "The cost of not looking at context," said Wakefield, "is you think anyone who comes under this diagnosis has a biological disorder, so should more or less automatically get antidepressant medication, and everything else is superfluous." His colleague Horwitz added, "There is a trend to treat people in this somewhat mechanized way. People are starting to think that any sort of negative emotion is unnatural, that they can take medication and feel better. What that can also do is make it less likely for people to make real changes in their lives that might be better than medications."

I'm no expert in psychiatric diagnosis, but on a commonsense basis, it looks like the two professors might have a good point. A new, revised version of the *DSM* is expected to be issued in 2011, and it will be interesting to see what happens to the definition of depression. In the meantime, there's a lot of money tied up in the existing definition (which I should stress is currently followed by the overwhelming majority of experts in the field): drug company profits, research funding, insurance reimbursements for doctors.

Here's another widely used screening test for depression. Let's see how you score:

QUICK DEPRESSION SELF-TEST

This is a widely used quick self-test for screening depression, called the Center for Epidemiologic Studies Depression Scale (CES-D).

It measures depressive feelings and behaviors over the last week. It is not meant to give you a clinical diagnosis, but as an exercise for you to gain information about your emotional health, and if necessary, to discuss with a mental health professional.

The twenty questions below refer to how you felt and acted *during the last week*. Check the appropriate statement.

Note: all questions need to be answered.

DURING THE LAST WEEK:

1. I was bothered by things that don't usually bother me.

Rarely or none of the time (<1 day) _____
Some or a little of the time (1–2 days) _____
Occasionally or a moderate amount of the time (3–4 days) _____
Most or all of the time (5–7 days) _____

2. I did not feel like eating; my appetite was poor.

Rarely or none of the time (<1 day) _____
Some or a little of the time (1–2 days) _____
Occasionally or a moderate amount of the time (3–4 days) _____
Most or all of the time (5–7 days) _____

3. I felt that I could not shake off the blues even with the help of my family or friends.

Rarely or none of the time (<1 day) _____
Some or a little of the time (1–2 days) _____
Occasionally or a moderate amount of the time (3–4 days) _____
Most or all of the time (5–7 days) _____

4. I felt that I was just as good as other people.

Rarely or none of the time (<1 day) _____
Some or a little of the time (1–2 days) _____
Occasionally or a moderate amount of the time (3–4 days) _____
Most or all of the time (5–7 days) _____

5. I had trouble keeping my mind on what I was doing.

Rarely or none of the time (<1 day) ____

Some or a little of the time (1–2 days) ____

Occasionally or a moderate amount of the time (3–4 days) ____

Most or all of the time (5–7 days) ____

6. I felt depressed.

Rarely or none of the time (<1 day) ____

Some or a little of the time (1–2 days) ____

Occasionally or a moderate amount of the time (3–4 days) ____

Most or all of the time (5–7 days) ____

7. I felt everything I did was an effort.

Rarely or none of the time (<1 day) ____

Some or a little of the time (1–2 days) ____

Occasionally or a moderate amount of the time (3–4 days) ____

Most or all of the time (5–7 days) ____

8. I felt hopeful about the future.

Rarely or none of the time (<1 day) ____

Some or a little of the time (1–2 days) ____

Occasionally or a moderate amount of the time (3–4 days) ____

Most or all of the time (5–7 days) ____

9. I thought my life had been a failure.

Rarely or none of the time (<1 day) ____

Some or a little of the time (1–2 days) ____

Occasionally or a moderate amount of the time (3–4 days) ____

Most or all of the time (5–7 days) ____

10. I felt fearful.

Rarely or none of the time (<1 day) _____

Some or a little of the time (1–2 days) _____

Occasionally or a moderate amount of the time (3–4 days) _____

Most or all of the time (5–7 days) _____

11. My sleep was restless.

Rarely or none of the time (<1 day) _____

Some or a little of the time (1–2 days) _____

Occasionally or a moderate amount of the time (3–4 days) _____

Most or all of the time (5–7 days) _____

12. I was happy.

Rarely or none of the time (<1 day) _____

Some or a little of the time (1–2 days) _____

Occasionally or a moderate amount of the time (3–4 days) _____

Most or all of the time (5–7 days) _____

13. I talked less than usual.

Rarely or none of the time (<1 day) _____

Some or a little of the time (1–2 days) _____

Occasionally or a moderate amount of the time (3–4 days) _____

Most or all of the time (5–7 days) _____

14. I felt lonely.

Rarely or none of the time (<1 day) _____

Some or a little of the time (1–2 days) _____

Occasionally or a moderate amount of the time (3–4 days) _____

Most or all of the time (5–7 days) _____

15. People were unfriendly.

Rarely or none of the time (<1 day) ____

Some or a little of the time (1–2 days) ____

Occasionally or a moderate amount of the time (3–4 days) ____

Most or all of the time (5–7 days) ____

16. I enjoyed life.

Rarely or none of the time (<1 day) ____

Some or a little of the time (1–2 days) ____

Occasionally or a moderate amount of the time (3–4 days) ____

Most or all of the time (5–7 days) ____

17. I had crying spells.

Rarely or none of the time (<1 day) ____

Some or a little of the time (1–2 days) ____

Occasionally or a moderate amount of the time (3–4 days) ____

Most or all of the time (5–7 days) ____

18. I felt sad.

Rarely or none of the time (<1 day) ____

Some or a little of the time (1–2 days) ____

Occasionally or a moderate amount of the time (3–4 days) ____

Most or all of the time (5–7 days) ____

19. I felt that people disliked me.

Rarely or none of the time (<1 day) ____

Some or a little of the time (1–2 days) ____

Occasionally or a moderate amount of the time (3–4 days) ____

Most or all of the time (5–7 days) ____

20. I could not get "going."

Rarely or none of the time (<1 day) _____

Some or a little of the time (1–2 days) _____

Occasionally or a moderate amount of the time (3–4 days) _____

Most or all of the time (5–7 days) _____

Using this chart, add up your score:

Scoring the Test

Item Weights	Rarely or none of the time (less than 1 day)	Some or a little of the time (1–2 days)	Occasionally or a moderate amount of the time (3–4 days)	Most or all of the time (5–7 days)
Items 4, 8, 12, & 16	3	2	1	0
All other Items:	0	1	2	3

A score of 16 or greater is considered depressed. If you score as depressed, see your doctor and/or a mental health professional.

This test is widely used by professionals and the general population, but no test is perfect, and you should consider this as an informational exercise to see how you score, and as a prelude, not a substitute, for professional help if necessary.

What does it mean for you?

If you're diagnosed with depression, I think you should make sure you fully understand the diagnosis, and discuss with your doctor/ psychiatrist whether you're experiencing normal human sadness.

THE BENEFITS OF HAPPINESS

Once we realize that a "life of happiness" will naturally include periods of stress, tragedy, sadness, and even depression, then the destination becomes clearer and more achievable.

I know in my soul that true happiness is real, it is possible, and it is achievable.

You and I should try to understand happiness, and pursue it with all our might. For one thing, it's really good for you!

In 2005–2008, a team of researchers at the University College London published some fascinating studies showing that, in a nutshell, happiness may help you live longer and healthier. It is some of the first research to demonstrate the effects of positive human emotions, especially happiness, on human physiology and the immune system. Among their findings:

- Emotions are intimately involved in the initiation or progression of cancer, HIV, cardiovascular disease, and autoimmune disorders. There is evidence to support the theory that people with more negative emotions have a weaker immune system and higher risk for illness than those with more positive emotions.
- Negative emotional states like depression are associated with premature death and increased risk of coronary heart disease, type 2 diabetes, and disability.
- Positive emotions are associated with better inflammatory and cardiovascular activity.

In the course of over twenty years of studying happiness and what he calls "subjective well-being," Professor Ed Diener at the University of Illinois has found that in general, happy people may be more successful in their careers and marriages, be more creative, be more resilient in tough situations, and have stronger social relationships than less happy people.

Happiness is good for the spirit, the mind, and the body. And it is a critical ingredient in living well.

I believe happiness is not only good for your health, it is your birthright.

Happiness is your destiny.

With the proper understanding and effort, you can find, nurture, and build your personal happiness.

HAPPINESS EXERCISE

One-Minute Life Satisfaction Test
How Satisfied Are You with Your Life?

This short test measures your overall satisfaction with your life.

It takes about a minute to complete.

Below are five statements that you may agree or disagree with.

Using the 1–7 scale below, indicate your agreement with each item by placing the appropriate number on the line before that item.

7 – Strongly agree

6 – Agree

5 – Slightly agree

4 – Neither agree nor disagree

3 – Slightly disagree

2 – Disagree

1 – Strongly disagree

___ In most ways my life is close to my ideal.

___ The conditions of my life are excellent.

___ I am satisfied with my life.

___ So far I have gotten the important things I want in life.

___ If I could live my life over, I would change almost nothing.

___ ADD UP TO TOTAL SCORE

1. If you scored 35–31: You are Extremely satisfied with your life.

2. If you scored 26–30: You are Satisfied with your life.

3. If you scored 21–25: You are Slightly satisfied with your life.

4. If you scored 20: Neutral

5. If you scored 15–19: You are Slightly dissatisfied with your life.

6. If you scored 10–14: You are Dissatisfied with your life.

7. If you scored 5–9: You are Extremely dissatisfied with your life.

Source: Ed Diener, Robert A. Emmons, Randy J. Larsen, and Sharon Griffin, "The Satisfaction with Life Scale," *Journal of Personality Assessment*, 1985, 49. For an in-depth discussion of the test results, go to: http://www.psych.uiuc.edu/~ediener/, then click on: "Research Information," then "Satisfaction with Life Scale," then "Understanding the SWLS Scores."

An Emotional Spectrum

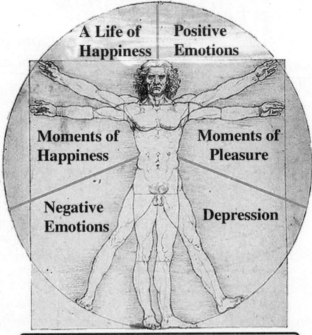

A Life of Happiness | Positive Emotions

Moments of Happiness | Moments of Pleasure

Negative Emotions | Depression

A LIFE OF HAPPINESS, LIVING WELL EMOTIONALLY

Fulfillment, life satisfaction, personal growth, meaning, emotional thriving, flourishing, love and joy over the long term, serving a greater good and stretching beyond yourself, in a life that also includes natural periods of sadness, sorrow and tragedy.

MOMENTS OF HAPPINESS

Emotional enjoyment and absorption: playing with your children, spending time with friends and family, enjoying a good book, gardening, hobbies.

MOMENTS OF PLEASURE

Physical gratifications like food, sex, music, laughter, exercise.

POSITIVE EMOTIONS

Love, joy, interest, contentment, gratitude, empathy, compassion, amusement, exhilaration, intrigue, excitement, wonder, tranquility, serenity, work satisfaction, pride in achievement.

NEGATIVE EMOTIONS

Negative rhythms of life: anger, failure, jealousy, embarrassment, fear, anxiety, stress, shame. Sadness and grief: natural human emotions in response to life events that can worsen into "unipolar depression," the most common psychological disorder.

DEPRESSION

An episodic or sustained mental disorder that causes impairment. A condition requiring professional help.

THE HAPPINESS FORMULA: THE SINGLE MOST IMPORTANT THING I HAVE LEARNED IN MY ENTIRE LIFE

Are you ready for this?

Here's the single most important thing I've learned in my entire life:

You alone are the person who owns the definition of who you are.

That one idea has been the guiding principle of my life.

I refuse to be defined by other people's limits, or their expectations, or their perceptions of me. As the English poet W. E. Henley wrote, "I am the master of my fate: I am the captain of my soul."

I believe you should print this idea in capital letters in your soul: I ALONE OWN THE DEFINITION OF WHO I AM!

Don't let anybody tell you what you can be or can't be. If you think it, believe it, and live it, I guarantee that you'll start down a path to transform your life and live better every single day.

This is especially true when it comes to your happiness and your emotional life.

Don't let anybody tell you how you should feel and what your emotions should be. You have the right to be as happy or as sad as you want to be, and you alone have the responsibility, and the power, to create your own happiness, nobody else.

In grade school, a teacher verbally beat me up for a mistake I'd made and turned it into a racial insult, saying, "You people will never amount to anything." She wanted to force her twisted, pathetic definition and warped worldview onto my soul. As a kid, I should have felt really sad, right? Well, I did. But that insult became a rallying cry for me to overachieve and outperform for the rest of my life, to pursue success and happiness on my terms, not hers.

Those seven words were a hell of a positive motivator for me. Maybe I should track that clown down and buy her a drink.

When I was starting my new TV talk show in 1990 and shopping it around to local affiliates, a bigmouthed TV station manager in Texas said in effect, "There's no way an unknown bald-headed black man is going to make it as a talk show host in America. And he's not going to make it in this market. Forget it!" He painted me like some kind of freak. His message to me was: "You can't." Oh, really? The second you tell me "I can't," I'm going to prove you wrong, dude. I don't plan to fail.

I don't believe in the word "no" when it comes to my success and happiness. I took that station manager's negative and flipped it into a positive. I hustled my butt off, put my heart and soul into that show, and got it on the air nationally for seventeen years, and won multiple Emmy Award nominations while entertaining and informing millions of people. I ran his definition of me right over.

In 1999, when the doctor told me I had multiple sclerosis, he told me in effect, "You can't continue your life. Go home and wait to die."

Rather than surrender my happiness at that moment, I decided to get a new team of doctors, and charge ahead with the business of fighting hard, feeling positive, and enjoying every second of life. Ten years later, I'm still charging ahead, all day, every day.

When you step into my office, you'll see a giant framed illustration that dominates the entire wall behind where I sit. It is a photograph of the climactic scene of the motion picture *Glory*. It depicts the moment when the proud, exhausted, fiercely determined 624 black soldiers of the 54th Massachusetts Volunteer Infantry Regiment began a charge up the shore of the Atlantic Ocean in the evening sun of July 18, 1863, toward the Confederate guns of Fort Wagner, their bayonets fixed in a wall of steel, charging into a maelstrom of smoke, flames, explosions, bullets, cannon fire, and pure chaos.

That photograph captures the essence of my life. And it captures the idea that rules my life: the reality that as the Roman emperor Marcus

Aurelius put it, "The whole universe is change and life itself is but what you deem it."

Life itself is but what you deem it. The great self-help guru Dale Carnegie considered those eight words as capable of transforming your life, and I agree.

It is not up to your boss to make you happy.

It is not your friend's job or your preacher's job and it's not up to your doctor or psychiatrist.

It is not even your family's job to make you happy.

It is all up to you! Life is what you deem it.

It's important to understand that happiness is something you do, not something you find.

In *Julius Caesar* William Shakespeare wrote, "There is a tide in the affairs of men, / Which, taken at the flood, leads on to fortune; / Omitted, all the voyage of their life / Is bound in shallows and in miseries." I believe that tide occurs every morning when you wake up and look at yourself in the mirror, and every hour, every second of your life. Every moment is a new opportunity to create happiness for yourself. As Psalm 118 puts it, "This is the day which the Lord hath made; we will rejoice and be glad in it."

You create your own life. You create your own happiness. You make the choice whether you are happy or unhappy. It's not the circumstances that force the happiness or unhappiness on you.

You determine your own emotional health. You determine your perceptions of the events that occur to you, and it's up to you to make them into positive emotions. As the poet John Milton argued, "The mind is its own place, and in itself can make a heaven of hell, a hell of heaven."

There are two powerful currents of thought that feed the truth of these insights. One school is the wisdom of the ages and the other is modern science.

TWO THOUSAND YEARS OF HAPPINESS WISDOM AGREES:

YOU ARE THE MASTER
OF YOUR OWN FATE.

AND YOU CREATE
YOUR OWN HAPPINESS.

Those two simple, powerful ideas are the two edges of the same sword, and they have echoed in the thoughts of great minds throughout time.

> *Happiness depends upon ourselves.*
>
> —ARISTOTLE

> *If I am not for myself, then who will be for me? And if I am only for myself, then what am I? And if not now, when?*
>
> —HILLEL THE ELDER, FIRST CENTURY BC

> *It's never the events that happen that make us disturbed, but our view of them.*
>
> —EPICTETUS, FIRST CENTURY AD

> *Happiness is life, and life is the fulfillment of action.*
>
> —ARIUS, FOURTH CENTURY AD

> *O mortal men, why seek ye for happiness abroad, when it is placed within yourselves?*
>
> —BOETHIUS, AD 520

> *Happiness and misery depend as much on temperament as on fortune.*
>
> —FRANCOIS DE LA ROCHEFOUCAULD, SEVENTEENTH CENTURY

Man is the artificer of his own happiness.
>—HENRY DAVID THOREAU, 1838

All happiness is in the mind.
>—HENRY G. BOHN, 1855

Most people are about as happy as they make up their minds to be.
>—ABRAHAM LINCOLN

Happiness does not depend on outward things, but on the way we see them.
>—LEO TOLSTOY

To be in hell is to drift; to be in heaven is to steer.
>—GEORGE BERNARD SHAW, 1903

It is not that someone else is preventing you from living happily; you yourself do not know what you want. Rather than admit this, you pretend that someone is keeping you from exercising your liberty. Who is this? It is yourself.
>—THOMAS MERTON, 1961

I am responsible for the achievement of my desires.
I am responsible for my choices and actions . . .
I am responsible for my personal happiness.
>—DR. NATHANIEL BRANDEN,
>PSYCHOLOGIST, AUTHORITY ON SELF-ESTEEM

I've been saying things like this for most of my adult life, when I've addressed audiences of thousands as a speaker, and when I stare at my own mug in the mirror in the morning.

The funny thing is that not only have these truths been celebrated by the world's best self-help gurus and biggest motivational speakers, from Norman Vincent Peale and Dale Carnegie to Tony Robbins and Les Brown—but now modern science is actually catching up with them!

And in recent history, science has made some astonishing breakthroughs to help us on the journey toward happiness.

CHAPTER 3

Seven Breakthroughs on the Road to Happiness

O ne day in January 2001, three psychology professors got together at a tropical resort in a small town in Mexico to think
about happiness.

They decided to try to tackle a cosmic question: what is the overall
"architecture" of human happiness?

They didn't have much good information to go on, as happiness research was still a very new field. Over the next few years, the professors
reviewed studies on twins raised together and apart, which provide intriguing clues to how happiness is inherited. They looked at studies of
the impact of wealth and marriage on people's emotional well-being.
They dug into surveys of well-being across different countries. They
reviewed hundreds of other studies, exchanging ideas and picking apart
the data.

The question that most intrigued them was, given strong evidence
that we are born with a genetically predetermined happiness "set point"
that stays fairly constant through our lives no matter what happens to
us, can we make ourselves permanently happier? Their conclusion? A
resounding yes.

Happiness Breakthrough #1:
The Happiness Formula

The three professors, Sonja Lyubomirsky, Ken Sheldon, and David Schkade, published their findings in 2005 and included a remarkable pie chart that illustrates their proposed formula for happiness, based on all the research to date. My summary of their conclusions:

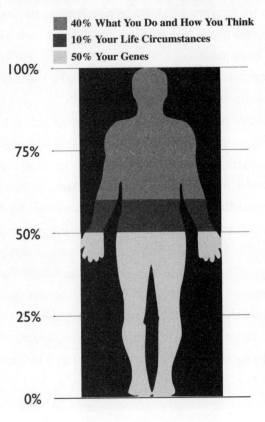

The Secret of Happiness

- 40% What You Do and How You Think
- 10% Your Life Circumstances
- 50% Your Genes

This is a thrilling intellectual breakthrough, and it has huge implications for your happiness.

At first glance, these rough estimates look kind of intimidating. The idea that, on average, our genes determine 50 percent of our happiness, locking in a genetic "set point" or "set range" of happiness, led another researcher to wisecrack that maybe "trying to be happier is like trying to be taller."

On top of that is the 10 percent determined by your life circumstances— your income, family dynamics, health, and the place you live—all of which can be changed, but usually not very easily or quickly. And even when life circumstances do change, the effect is temporary; research on both paraplegics and lottery winners suggests that on average, a year after these dramatic changes in their circumstances, they gravitated back to their original set ranges of happiness anyway. "Once you get basic human needs met, a lot more money doesn't make a lot more happiness," reported Dan Gilbert, a psychology professor at Harvard University. It can take longer to rebound from the loss of a job or a loved one, but we still seem to settle back to the genetically determined set range.

But look at the 40 percent element of the equation, which Lyubomirsky, Sheldon, and Schkade called "daily intentional activities." A huge slice of happiness, it turns out, is *directly in our control*. It is governed by the voluntary actions we take every day, by the things we do and the attitudes we take. "We're not slaves to our genes," said Lyubomirsky, "and we don't have to wait for someone else to do something good to make us feel better."

This insight validates what the greatest minds of history have been telling us for over two thousand years, and what I've always believed: *You can control your own happiness.* You are the master of your own fate, and you create your own happiness, by how you think and what you do.

❧ *Happiness is something you can work at. It's a matter of identifying the things you do that get in the way of happiness, and figuring out what positive activities you can do every day to augment it.*

—PROFESSOR DAVID LYKKEN, UNIVERSITY OF MINNESOTA

HAPPINESS TIPS

Eight Habits of the Happiest People: What They Do and How They Think

What, then, should we do, and how should we think, to be happier?

"If you want to keep your happiness at the higher end of the set range," Professor Lyubomirsky told a reporter for *US News & World Report,* "you have to commit yourself every day to doing things to make you happy." She and other experts have noticed some fascinating patterns emerge among the happiest people they've examined in their studies. These people tend to:

- **Deeply enjoy and nurture relationships** with family and friends.
- **Be grateful** for everything life offers.
- **Think positively and optimistically** about life events and about the future.
- **Commit strongly** to life goals.
- **Be generous and forgiving** with other people.
- **Be self-confident and resilient** in the face of stress and tragedy.
- **Savor life's pleasures** and live "in the moment."
- **Be physically active on a regular basis,** even every day.

LIVING WELL EMOTIONALLY EXPERT
Dr. Sonja Lyubomirsky

Sonja Lyubomirsky, Ph.D., is Professor of Psychology at the University of California, Riverside. Originally from Russia, she received her AB, summa cum laude, from Harvard University and her Ph.D. in social/personality psychology from Stanford University. Lyubomirsky currently teaches courses in social psychology and positive psychology and serves as the Department of Psychology's graduate advisor. Her teaching and mentoring of students have been recognized with the Faculty of the Year and Faculty Mentor of the Year awards.

In 2002, Lyubomirsky was awarded a Templeton Positive Psychology Prize. Currently, she is an associate editor of the Journal of Positive Psychology *and (with Ken Sheldon) holds a five-year million-dollar grant from the National Institute of Mental Health to conduct research on the possibility of permanently increasing happiness.*

In her work, Lyubomirsky has focused on developing a science of human happiness. To this end, her research addresses three critical questions: (1) What makes people happy? (2) Is happiness a good thing? and (3) How can we make people happier still? She is currently exploring the potential of happiness-sustaining activities—for example, expressing gratitude, doing acts of kindness, visualizing one's "best possible selves," and reflecting on happy moments—to durably increase a person's happiness level. She has been conducting research on happiness for eighteen years and has published widely in the area.

Some people think that if happiness is influenced by genetics, then there's nothing you can do about your happiness.

Then there are people who don't make as much money as they want,

(continued)

or live in a place they don't want to live in, and they think that's going to doom them to a life of unhappiness.

But that's not true. Of course genetics and life circumstances affect your happiness, but up to 40 percent is affected by your intentional, purposeful, conscious effort.

This doesn't mean it's easy to become happier. Happiness-building behaviors can sometimes be hard to enact, just as losing weight isn't that easy. If you're not a generally happy person, it may be hard for you to change your habits and start looking at things in a more optimistic way, or be more grateful.

A theme that runs through my book and my research is that it can take a lot of effort, especially at the beginning, but once you start to develop good habits, it will become easier over time.

There are a lot of happiness books out there, and most are based on people's intuition, or anecdotes, or on personal experiences and observations that are all interesting and valid in and of themselves.

But I wanted to take a more scientific approach. If you're going to take a new drug, wouldn't you want to make sure that it's been tested in randomized controlled studies, not just because your friend told you it's going to work? It's the same thing with happiness.

I'm generally a pretty happy person. I'm not really "high," but I'm moderately happy and generally optimistic. I usually see the positive side of life. I look forward to the future and I feel like I have something to look forward to. In my own life, I've started doing more of some happiness-building strategies that I wasn't as good at in the past.

For example, one strategy is to live more in the present moment and savor it. I'm usually really busy and future-oriented. But when I'm with my seven- and nine-year-old children now, I've really been trying to enjoy the moment more, and not worry about what I'm doing tomorrow.

For me, exercise gives me real fulfillment. It boosts mood, and it's also a goal that you can shoot for and achieve regularly. There are data showing that exercise makes people feel happier.

It's really important to choose your "happiness strategies" wisely. Not every strategy will be beneficial for every person. It's going to differ, based on what your natural strengths are. For some people it's expressing gratitude, for others it may be focusing on their goals, or being more forgiving. It's going to depend on the person, which is why I include a diagnostic test in my book *The How of Happiness* to help people identify which strategy is going to work better for them.

I get hundreds of e-mails, including from people who tell me the book changed their lives. One of my favorites is from a guy who said he'd read lots of self-help books, but they never really worked. He would get all excited and try all these different strategies, and then get overwhelmed and stop doing them. But he took our test to determine the four top activities that he should try first. And for the first time in his life, he's gotten happier in a way he's been able to maintain, because he's taking it one step at a time. ⋘

Happiness Breakthrough #2:
The New Talk Therapy

Have you ever been in therapy?

If you haven't, and the only frame of reference you've got is *The Sopranos* or old Woody Allen movies, I wouldn't blame you for being skeptical. But that's the old-fashioned kind of psychotherapy.

There's a really exciting kind of therapy you may not know about. It can really help you if you need it. When it's done right, it can be a tremendously effective tool for living a more rewarding emotional life and breaking through to happiness.

It all started one day about a half century ago, when a short blue-eyed man in a bow tie sat in his office at the University of Pennsylvania and thought about Sigmund Freud.

The man was Aaron Beck, a doctor and psychiatrist, and the thought process he began that day would eventually shake the pillars of psychology, and transform him into a figure who today is revered by some in his profession as even bigger and better than the man who invented modern psychiatry decades earlier, Freud himself.

On that day, Aaron Beck started figuring out a new way of making people feel happier.

Some of Sigmund Freud's ideas still hold up very well. He identified the importance of the unconscious mind. He saw that childhood experiences can shape adult emotions. And perhaps most important, he pioneered the idea that people with mental and emotional problems can improve themselves by talking to a trained listener—a therapist. "Talk therapy" was born.

But it turns out Freud got a lot of things wrong. He largely misunderstood female psychology. He placed way too much emphasis on childhood repressed memories, dreams, the Oedipus complex, and penis envy. And many experts came to believe that the Freudian method of talk therapy didn't seem to work all that well.

Dr. Beck, who was trained in Freudian principles of psychotherapy, was especially frustrated by having to listen to his depressed patients drone on and on as they lay on his couch for months or years on end, rehashing their problems and making little progress. "The idea was that if you sat back and listened and said 'Aha,' somehow secrets would come out," Beck told the *New York Times*. "And you would get exhausted just from the helplessness of it."

So slowly, Dr. Beck broke free of Freud, applied major tweaks to the process of talk therapy, and created a new form that has come to be called "cognitive therapy," or "cognitive behavioral therapy" (CBT).

Beck got his patients up off his couch and talked to them face-to-face.

He helped patients identify and correct negative "automatic thoughts" about themselves, the world, and the future.

Rather than focus heavily on childhood trauma, parental failings, or dreams, Beck and his patients concentrated on the here and now, and collaborated on tackling what Beck called "commonsense problems that people have." He gave his patients "homework" assignments to correct distorted beliefs, promote healthy thinking, and improve their behavior. He gave them positive reinforcement, and encouraged them to schedule life-enhancing, pleasurable activities into their routines.

And Dr. Beck noticed something beautiful starting to happen.

Rather than spending years being stuck in their problems, Dr. Beck's depressed patients often got better quickly, sometimes in as little as a few weeks of therapy.

> ☙ Depressed people are caught in a feedback loop in which distorted thoughts cause negative feelings, which then distort thinking further.
>
> You can break the cycle by changing the thoughts.
>
> A big part of cognitive therapy is training clients to catch the thoughts and distortions and then find alternative and more accurate ways of thinking.
>
> Over many weeks, the client's thoughts become more realistic. The feedback loop is broken and the client's anxiety or depression abates.
>
> —JONATHAN HAIDT, PSYCHOLOGIST AND HAPPINESS RESEARCHER

Dr. Beck completely revolutionized and improved talk therapy, and remade it into a powerhouse tool for getting people on the road to a happier life.

Today it is widely considered among the most effective forms of nondrug treatment for depression, and has also proven effective for treating anxiety, addictions, panic attacks, and eating disorders.

Today, Beck's cognitive therapy is considered one of the most researched and most effective forms of psychotherapy for mild and moderate depression, anxiety, and obsessive-compulsive disorders, and is also considered effective for severe depression in combination with medication.

Insurance companies and managed-care companies love cognitive therapy because it works—and in weeks or months instead of years. Unfortunately, as the *Washington Post* noted, since "few academics or private psychiatrists have the ad budgets of, say, Eli Lilly, the public remains largely unaware of the research supporting the efficacy of cognitive therapy or other talking cures."

Remember Tony Soprano's psychiatrist, Dr. Melfi? Dr. Beck says she got it all wrong.

"She was just following the old road—it's all due to his mother," argued Beck, "rather than getting from him what he feels and thinks." Beck thinks he could have solved Tony's panic attacks in just a few sessions. Rather than keeping Tony in old-fashioned psychotherapy for year after year rehashing his dysfunctional childhood and his dreams, Beck says he and Tony would have collaborated on setting up goals for the short term, then mapped out new behaviors to achieve the goals.

Another talk therapy that gets good results for depression is called interpersonal therapy, a highly practical short-term approach that helps people deal with grief, relationship problems, and life changes.

What's the bottom line? Talk therapy works, and if you think you could benefit from it, cognitive therapy and interpersonal therapy are tools you should look into and discuss with your doctor.

Remember that any therapy is only as good as the therapist who uses it, so choose one wisely and one with whom you feel very comfortable. "A degree in psychiatry or psychology is no guarantee of genius," wrote Andrew Solomon in his book *The Noonday Demon*, adding that you should "use the utmost care in choosing a psychiatrist," since you are literally "placing your mind in the hands of this person."

LIVING WELL EMOTIONALLY EXPERT
Dr. Richard Rosenthal

Dr. Richard N. Rosenthal is Chairman of Psychiatry at St. Luke's Roosevelt Hospital Center, New York, and Professor of Clinical Psychiatry at Columbia University. He is also Past President of the American Academy of Addiction Psychiatry, a Distinguished Fellow of the American Psychiatric Association, and a Fellow of the New York Academy of Medicine.

He is a diplomate of the American Board of Psychiatry and Neurology in psychiatry, with subspecialty certification in addiction psychiatry. Previously, he was associate chairman for psychiatric clinical services of Beth Israel Medical Center, New York, and directed the division on substance abuse at Albert Einstein College of Medicine.

He maintains a private practice of psychotherapy and psychopharmacology for mood and addictive disorders. Dr. Rosenthal is among New York Magazine's *"Best Doctors" for 2008.*

Dr. Rosenthal's main research focus has been on the evaluation and treatment of the severely mentally ill with co-occurring addictive disorders, and he has been a clinical, research, and program development consultant to hospitals, state and federal agencies, and the pharmaceutical industry.

(continued)

If you're feeling bad emotionally, but you're not obviously stricken with a severe mental illness, our culture tends to say, "Buck up, pull yourself up by your bootstraps."

Some critics argue that we overmedicalize emotional problems and that we've turned low moods, such as mourning, into a disease. I don't disagree with that; I agree people can have normal low moods and I think we need to be skeptical. On the other hand, some of us have real depression. A person may be suffering needlessly from a real disorder and suffering real impairment.

If, for example, several months after losing a loved one or another stressful event you're still impaired, you may need help. You may be functioning poorly at school or work. You're not eating properly, you've lost weight, you feel guilty, your motivation has gone out the window, you can't concentrate, you're not taking pleasure in normal daily activities and relationships and you have a reduction in your sex drive. Then you may have a real depression.

It makes sense to think about whether the pain you're experiencing has value. You can experience emotional and psychological and spiritual growth when you navigate your way through pain. But on the other hand, if you're not getting that value, maybe you need help getting that value, and maybe that pain doesn't have to be as large or as constant as you are experiencing it.

People should not suffer needlessly. We can learn from certain kinds of pain: you put your hand on a hot burner, and it teaches you something. But there are other kinds of pain, emotional pain, that perhaps you need somebody to work with on: someone from your faith, or a professional mental health provider.

When you talk with an objective expert like a therapist, somebody who is really on your side, you can discover patterns in problems. It's been helpful in my life, as a patient. I found it very valuable. There were things about myself that I was either ignoring or unaware of, that were getting in my way.

We all have this belief that we know ourselves. The problem is that there is a lot that we hide from ourselves that's uncomfortable or painful or frightening or threatening.

If you work with a compassionate therapist, you'll soon realize that he or she is really on your team. This person's job is to be in your corner. Sometimes that means telling you unpleasant truths about yourself so you can wise up about them—so you can grow.

If you have severe depression, you probably need medication. That's what the evidence says. But for mild-to-moderate depression, cognitive therapy works pretty well. It works on your "thought generator," the part of your mind that generates depressive thoughts and negative feedback. Cognitive behavioral therapy [CBT] helps you be aware of and amenable to positive feedback from your environment, which allows your thinking and your behavior to improve.

The thing that's nice about CBT is that it's a skill set for you to learn, techniques to navigate stressful or negative situations that become a part of your behavioral "toolbox." In fact, many different studies show that six months to a year after the end of therapy, people are still using those tools effectively. So it really works.

When you decide to take responsibility for your emotional life, it can be painful or scary when you take that first step. But it's a courageous step, which will ultimately empower you.

It takes courage to get help, and to look at yourself and face the issues that you've avoided for years. That courage can have a very positive value in your life.

If you summon the courage to really look at yourself, the payoff is better

(continued)

awareness of yourself and a more truthful and more honest capacity to see who you really are in the real world.

And as a result, you'll make better choices about what's going to make you really happy. ఞ

Happiness Breakthrough #3:
Antidepressant Medication

I know people who have enjoyed near miracles in living well emotionally with the help of antidepressant medications.

And I know experts who warn us to be extremely cautious about the risks and side effects of antidepressants, including in the worst case, suicidal thinking, especially among younger people.

Right now, tens of millions of Americans are being treated with antidepressant medications like Prozac and other SSRIs (selective serotonin reuptake inhibitors).

Do Prozac and these other drugs work? For many people, absolutely. They need them and should get them. How do they work? Experts aren't really sure, other than having a balancing effect on brain chemicals called neurotransmitters and easing the symptoms of depression.

In this way, they have become a pathway for many depressed people, especially the severely depressed, to feel better and start moving toward a happier life. In particular, Prozac, the top-selling antidepressant, has been the subject of a huge amount of public and media attention, with national debates raging over its effectiveness, side effects, and possible dangers.

According to the National Institute for Mental Health, Prozac and other SSRIs are "generally safe and reliable," but some studies show they may have unintentional effects, especially on young people. In 2004, a U.S. Food and Drug Administration (FDA) review of data from studies involving nearly forty-four hundred children and teen-agers being treated for depression found that 4 percent of those who took antidepressants thought about or attempted suicide (although no suicides occurred), compared to 2 percent of those who took a placebo.

Critics say that Prozac is overprescribed, and that too many primary care doctors routinely dispense it for light or mild forms of depression, when it is most appropriate for severe depression. In the absence of effective psychotherapy, the criticism goes, this kind of drug-induced "artificial happiness" is counterproductive because it causes lightly or moderately depressed people to avoid the hard work of addressing their emotional problems by relying on a pill instead.

In 2008, a major study was published in *PLoS Medicine*, a respected journal published by the nonprofit Public Library of Science, that disputed the effectiveness of Prozac and three other new-generation antidepressants. The researchers crunched data from all the clinical trials submitted to the U.S. Food and Drug Administration in the licensing applications for the medications. They reported that, compared with a placebo (sugar pill), the medications "do not produce clinically significant improvements in depression in patients who initially have moderate or even very severe depression, but show significant effects only in the most severely depressed patients." They concluded that "there is little reason to prescribe new-generation antidepressant medications to any but the most severely depressed patients unless alternative treatments have been ineffective."

But a great many psychiatrists and primary care doctors and, most important, patients have reported lasting and even life-changing positive effects on patients' moods from the medications, changes that enable a great many patients to tackle their problems, ideally in conjunction with help from a therapist.

I believe that people have a right to feel sad and even a right to be depressed on occasion. We should absorb it as a part of who we are. But it doesn't have to define who we are, and we shouldn't suffer needlessly. I give full credit to the doctors who properly prescribe medications, and to the patients who take them, since there are people who are helped by them. At the same time there are people who also need therapy and even hospitalization for their emotional and mental challenges.

Where do I stand on antidepressants? I had a bad experience with one type of antidepressant, but that's one anecdote, about one drug, from one person. You're the expert on yourself, and you should grill your doctor about any medication. You should know all the facts, all the risks and benefits of any drug, including antidepressants, and decide what you should do for yourself, in consultation with your doctor and psychiatrist.

LIVING WELL EMOTIONALLY EXPERT
Dr. Joseph Glenmullen

Joseph Glenmullen, M.D., is a clinical instructor in psychiatry at Harvard Medical School, is on the staff of Harvard University Health Services, and is in private practice in Harvard Square.

He is a leading critic of what he considers to be the overuse of medication to treat mental and emotional conditions.

He is Board Certified in Psychiatry by the American Board of Psychiatry and Neurology, and is the author of two books on the side effects of antidepressants: Prozac Backlash *and* The Antidepressant Solution.

He has given expert testimony in over two dozen state and federal cases and to the U.S. Congress regarding the side effects of psychiatric drugs.

'm not antidrug—I prescribe antidepressant drugs—but I'm an advocate for patients to get information about their effectiveness and risks.

If you've got a severe condition, you really should consider an antidepressant, at least at the beginning of treatment, in conjunction with some kind of therapy to address your underlying issues. Your goal could be to get off the medication in a year or two, once you address the underlying problems.

But I don't think that antidepressants should be recommended to people with mild conditions. The other forms of treatment, like cognitive behavioral therapy, are more effective and more lasting. Unfortunately, a majority of people who are diagnosed with mild depression are prescribed antidepressants, because the distinction isn't made between mild depression and severe depression.

In the middle there's a gray zone of moderate depression, and then it's really the patient's call, as long as he is well informed.

Antidepressants are overprescribed, and patients are not warned enough about the potential side effects. We now have all these warnings that antidepressants can make people suicidal. And we also have more data on their effectiveness not being as great as people once thought. In many instances, they're not a whole lot better than a placebo, or sugar pills.

I'm not saying that the drugs shouldn't be used, but they should be used carefully and only when necessary. And patients should always be fully educated about the risks and the benefits and the alternatives. You should be as skeptical and informed as possible.

It's important that you get a thorough evaluation from a doctor, who spends at least forty-five minutes to an hour with you, not ten minutes. If you walk into your primary care doctor or your gynecologist's office and say, "I'm a little stressed out by how hectic my life is," be cautious if he

(continued)

immediately pulls out a prescription pad and says, "How about a little Prozac?" You really need to be cautious, even if you love your doctor. You might want to say, "How about we get a more thorough evaluation here, like from a psychiatrist?" We should take this a little more seriously.

Primary care doctors are under a lot of pressure from the managed-care insurers. They are under pressure not to refer their patients to specialists, and they're under pressure to see people for only ten or fifteen minutes. They're used to giving, for example, a year's worth of refills on your blood pressure pill or your arthritis pill and they're under pressure from the insurance companies to do the same with antidepressants. And that's not appropriate. People need more information, more frequent contact with the doctor, and more frequent monitoring.

It's important to recognize that diagnoses in psychiatry are very subjective. We don't have a single blood test or urine test or CAT scan to objectively diagnose psychiatric conditions; and the diagnostic criteria change over time. Also, the marketing of psychiatric drugs has resulted in expanding diagnoses to capture more people.

Recently, for example, the antidepressant drug Paxil has been marketed as a medication for "social anxiety disorder," which used to be called "social phobia." This used to be considered a very severe, very debilitating and rare condition. A psychiatrist might see a handful of cases in a lifetime. But the drug companies helped expand the definition through direct-to-consumer marketing so it now includes virtually anybody who is shy! It went from a rare condition to being an alleged epidemic.

It's important to educate yourself on all these drugs and not to make decisions on your own but jointly with your doctor.

Antidepressants should not be handed out like candy. They should be used carefully and only when necessary. ∾

Happiness Breakthrough #4:
Psychology Goes Positive

As I've thought about living well emotionally over the years, and tried to achieve it in my own life, I've always been struck by a terrible contradiction.

There's an entire profession—actually two professions, psychiatry and psychology—geared toward trying to help us understand and solve problems and help us feel better. But they seem to spend most of their time on figuring out how to *help sick people feel less sick instead.* There's a huge difference. Ever since Freud announced in the 1890s that the goal of therapy was to transform "hysterical misery" into "ordinary unhappiness," it seems the profession has been dominated by these low expectations.

There's this huge gap—it's like they've set the bar way too low and totally forgotten the other half of the equation: how to help us to feel positive, to thrive and flourish. They seem stuck in the Dark Ages.

I don't want to feel less terrible emotionally—I want to feel fantastic!

The reason you see tens of thousands of people flock to see religious leaders like Joel Osteen or motivational speakers like Tony Robbins is that they are yearning for positive messages. And some of the greatest wisdom on positive thinking has come from people having nothing to do with psychiatry or psychology.

One day in the late 1990s, that started to change, when a grumpy psychologist was confronted by his five-year-old daughter in their garden.

She was running around the grass having a great time, singing, dancing, and throwing weeds in the air. So the psychologist, a man named Martin Seligman, did what grumps do. He scolded her for interrupting his work.

His daughter, fed up with his attitude, asked him, "Why can't you stop being such a grouch?"

Seligman experienced a revelation. For years he'd been walking around like a dreary wet cloud in a family filled with sunshine. Soon he thought of his profession the same way. "I realized that my profession was half-baked," he recalled. "It wasn't enough for us to nullify disabling conditions and get to zero. We needed to ask, What are the enabling conditions that make human beings flourish?"

Before World War II, Seligman reasoned, one of the main jobs of psychology was to "make relatively untroubled people happier." But this was forgotten after the war, because most of the federal funding and research went to treating mental disorders like depression, anxiety, neurosis, delusions, paranoia, and obsessions. "We've forgotten about the rest of our mission as psychologists," Seligman explained to one conference. "Approximately thirty percent of people in the USA suffer from a severe mental disorder at one time or another. And we have done an excellent job of helping that thirty percent. It is now time to turn to the other seventy percent."

For years, Seligman had been researching what he called "learned helplessness," the self-defeating process of catastrophic thinking that can spiral into depression. He developed a process called "learned optimism" that taught people how to recognize negative thoughts and to realistically dispute them.

The field of psychology, Seligman realized, needed to be challenged in a similar way.

Like a man possessed by a great vision, Seligman set out to transform his profession. He launched a movement called positive psychology. And he's made quite an impact. In the last ten years Seligman and his colleagues at the University of Pennsylvania have created a growing specialty, complete with its own studies, scholarly journals, handbooks, and master's degrees, all of which are devoted to the study of positive emotion, positive character, and positive institutions.

A big part of positive psychology is conducting scientific, evidence-based research to find answers to the question, what can we do to be happier?

One of Professor Seligman's most interesting ideas is how he sees three roads to happiness, which I'll summarize this way:

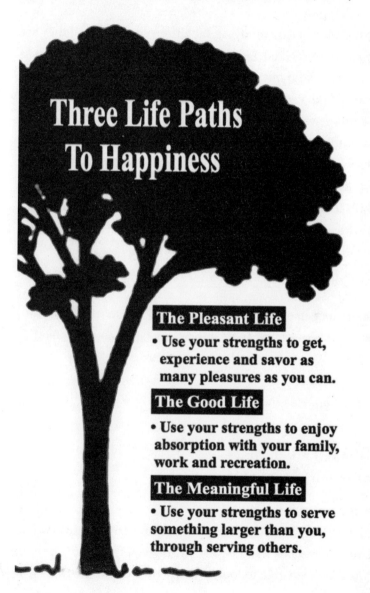

Three Life Paths To Happiness

The Pleasant Life
- Use your strengths to get, experience and savor as many pleasures as you can.

The Good Life
- Use your strengths to enjoy absorption with your family, work and recreation.

The Meaningful Life
- Use your strengths to serve something larger than you, through serving others.

There's nothing wrong with a taste of the Pleasant Life, but Americans have been oversold on it. We chase after the latest car or the best new flat-panel TV and think it will make us happier. But when we get them, the effect wears off quickly and we crave more material things. That's not true happiness.

Positive psychologists are studying the different paths, and they see deeper promise in the Good Life and the Meaningful Life. "This is newsworthy because so many Americans build their lives around pursuing pleasure," said Professor Seligman. "It turns out that engagement and meaning are much more important."

To me, a combination of the Good Life and the Meaningful Life is the most satisfying path to happiness, with moments of the Pleasant Life scattered through the days. I can think of nothing happier than to use all my skills to be totally engaged with my loved ones, my work, and my hobbies, while I strive to serve others.

HAPPINESS TIP

You can learn about the latest insights and breakthroughs of positive psychology, and take a number of happiness-related tests, by going to the excellent Web site maintained by Professor Martin Seligman and his colleagues:

www.authentichappiness.com

Happiness Breakthrough #5:
The Strengths and Virtues of Happiness

God has blessed me with the gift of gab.

I've been given the gift of the ability to speak on any topic anywhere in the world in five seconds flat. I've also been given the gift of strength of observation. I've been able to look into the lives of twenty-two thousand people over the course of seventeen years on my show and understand both the good and the bad that people are capable of.

I also have a very solid gift of persuasion. You could call it salesmanship. I have the ability to bring people together in a common cause, to present ideas and plans and have people buy into them. Sometimes I'll pitch a million-dollar idea in a business meeting and people will say yes even before they realize why they did! I've also got a mind like a computer, enabling me to pull up and analyze lots of different files simultaneously.

We all have strengths and virtues, and one of the keys to happiness is identifying specifically what your "Signature Strengths" are, and figuring out ways to exercise and enjoy them as much as you can in your daily life. I'm very lucky since I've been able to do that for most of my career.

A few years ago, a team of positive psychology researchers led by Martin Seligman and Professor Christopher Peterson at the University of Michigan decided to try to identify the human virtues and strengths that make life worth living, and give life purpose and meaning.

They analyzed three thousand years of wisdom on the subject: Buddhism, Hinduism, Confucianism, Christianity, Hebrew, and Islamic texts, the writings of Plato, Aristotle, and Aquinas. They were surprised to discover that six core virtues emerged consistently across different nations, cultures, and religions.

To me, all these virtues and strengths are equally valuable in achieving happiness. They all work together and multiply each other's power.

In my life, courage has been a hugely important virtue to draw on. For me, courage includes the power of positive thinking and the art of motivating yourself every single day to get the most out of life. The flip side of it is resilience, the ability to be able to absorb defeats, failures, and even disasters, and emerge a stronger, wiser person.

VIRTUES AND STRENGTHS THAT HELP YOU THRIVE

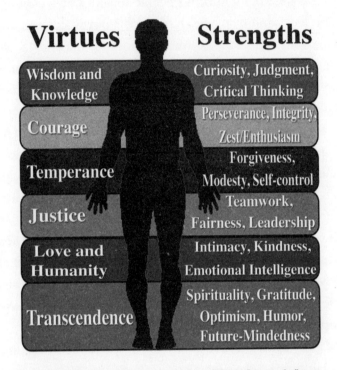

Virtues	Strengths
Wisdom and Knowledge	Curiosity, Judgment, Critical Thinking
Courage	Perseverance, Integrity, Zest/Enthusiasm
Temperance	Forgiveness, Modesty, Self-control
Justice	Teamwork, Fairness, Leadership
Love and Humanity	Intimacy, Kindness, Emotional Intelligence
Transcendence	Spirituality, Gratitude, Optimism, Humor, Future-Mindedness

Source: adapted from the work of Professors Martin Seligman, Christopher Peterson and colleagues

Remember Harold Dennis, the young man I told you about who was in the worst drunk driving accident in U.S. history?

He's a profile in raw courage if ever there was one. I mean, honestly, no matter what challenges the world threw at Harold, he fought back to overcome them. Some people let challenges like these take control of their lives, and other people fight back. That's Harold, all the way.

His school bus exploded and twenty-seven people died. Harold was horribly burned over much of his body, including his face.

His burns were so severe that his doctors ordered his nurses: "He's only fourteen. Don't let him look in a mirror. He's not ready.

He's not ready to endure the magnitude of his scars, so don't show him yet."

But Harold persuaded a nurse to slip him a mirror, and he experienced a moment he'd never forget. He couldn't recognize his own face. "Who's going to accept me?" he thought. "Friends, females? How is my life going to be now?"

Then, soon, another thought presented itself: "This is me. This is the new me. Figure out what to do."

Harold threw himself back into life, made the most of what he had, and pursued happiness on his own terms. He played soccer with a vengeance, which helped him refocus his life and perceive a clear path forward. He got a full scholarship to the University of Kentucky. He fought his way relentlessly onto the football team.

Although he once wondered whether a woman would ever go out with him, Harold met and married a beautiful lady named Donna. "He's so confident," she recalled. "He's such a confident person. You know, obviously, I see the scars. Everybody sees the scars. Or that's what I saw initially. But as soon as he speaks to you and you just see his confidence, I mean, it's just overwhelming."

And then, well, I'll let Harold finish the story:

> We have three kids. They're everything to me. I own my own development and construction management company. I knew that I would find happiness eventually.
>
> If I could go back and turn the hands of time and change course, I wouldn't do it. I wouldn't do it. I've endured and learned too much. Life's pretty good. Life's pretty good right now!

At the heart of courage is the belief in yourself, what some experts call "self-efficacy." The Stanford University psychologist Albert Bandura explained, "People need to learn how to manage failure so it's informational and not demoralizing."

*   *   *

Whenever you think you can't achieve something in the face of failure and adversity, you should remember these great moments in self-efficacy, and these motivational tips from some of the masters of history:

- Thomas Edison tried a thousand times before he could figure out how to make a lightbulb work properly.
- Walt Disney was canned by one boss who accused him of "lacking imagination."
- Decca Records blew off the Beatles when they were looking for a contract, declaring, "We don't like their sound."
- Steve Jobs and Steve Wozniak were blown off by both Hewlett-Packard and Atari when they pitched them a prototype of their first Apple computer.
- J. K. Rowling was rejected by almost every decent book company in London before her first Harry Potter book was acquired by a small publisher.
- Michael Jordan was cut from his high school basketball team.

MOTIVATION TIPS FROM THE MASTERS

Every day is a new life to a wise man.

—ANONYMOUS

If ye have faith as a grain of mustard seed, ye shall say unto this mountain, / Remove hence to yonder place; and it shall remove; and nothing shall be impossible unto you.

—MATTHEW 17:20

Have no anxiety about the morrow.

—JESUS

Our greatest glory is not in never falling, but in rising every time we fall.

—Confucius

Happy the Man, and happy he alone,
He who can call today his own:
He who, secure within, can say:
Tomorrow do thy worst, for I have lived today.

—Horace, Roman poet

Whether you think that you can or you can't, you're usually right.

—Henry Ford

For failure comes from the inside first,
It's there if we only knew it,
And you can win, though you face the worst,
If you feel that you're going to do it.

—Edgar A. Guest

For every day I stand outside your door,
And bid you wake, and rise to fight and win.
Wail not for precious chances passed away,
Weep not for golden ages on the wane!
Each night I burn the records of the day—
At sunrise every soul is born again!

—Walter Malone, "Opportunity"

Finish each day and be done with it. You have done what you could. Some blunders and absurdities no doubt have crept in; forget them as soon as you can.

Tomorrow is a new day; begin it well and serenely and with too high a spirit to be encumbered with your old nonsense.

—Ralph Waldo Emerson

Success begins with a fellow's will.
It's all in the state of mind.
If you think you are outclassed, you are,
You've got to think high to rise.
You've got to be sure of yourself before
You can ever win a prize.
Life's battles don't always go
To the stronger or faster man.
But soon or late the man who wins
Is the man who thinks he can.

—C. W. LONGENECKER, "THE VICTOR"

Courage is rightly esteemed as the first of human qualities because it is the quality which guarantees all others.

—WINSTON CHURCHILL

Action may not always bring happiness, but there is no happiness without action.

—BENJAMIN DISRAELI

The secret of being miserable is to have the leisure to bother about whether you are happy or not.

—GEORGE BERNARD SHAW

It is not how much we have but how much we enjoy that makes happiness.

—CHARLES H. SPURGEON

The secret of happiness is not in doing what one likes, but in liking what one has to do.

—JAMES M. BARRIE

To improve the golden moment of opportunity and catch the good that is within our reach is the great art of life.

—SAMUEL JOHNSON

The principle of happiness should be like the principle of virtue: it should not be dependent on things, but be a part of personality.

—WILLIAM LYON PHELPS

They can conquer who believe they can. He has not learned the first lesson of life who does not every day surmount a fear.

—RALPH WALDO EMERSON

Don't sweat the stupid stuff.

—MY FATHER, HERMAN WILLIAMS

The road to failure is paved with negativity. If you think you can't do something, chances are you won't be able to. Conversely, the power of positive thinking can turn an adverse situation into a prime opportunity for heroism.

—TIGER WOODS

I've failed over and over and over again in my life. That's why I succeed.

—MICHAEL JORDAN

LIVING WELL EMOTIONALLY EXPERT
Professor Christopher Peterson

Christopher Peterson, Ph.D., is Professor of Psychology and former Director of Clinical Training at the University of Michigan.

He is one of the world's leading researchers on positive psychology, optimism, well-being, and the connections between character strengths and happiness.

Professor Peterson is a member of the Positive Psychology Steering Committee; a consulting editor to the Journal of Positive Psychology; *a coeditor of* Health and Well-Being; *and a former Templeton Senior Fellow at the Positive Psychology Center of the University of Pennsylvania.*

He also holds an appointment as an Arthur F. Thurnau Professor at the University of Michigan, in recognition of his contributions to teaching. His most recent book is A Primer in Positive Psychology, *published in 2006.*

We developed a list of twenty-four different character strengths, and then we did a number of studies looking at how those character strengths relate to happiness and life satisfaction.

We find that among adults there are five strengths in particular that are big predictors of how happy or satisfied somebody is. I tell people, if you do any of these things well, then you should do more of them. The five strengths are:

- optimism
- curiosity
- gratitude

- zest/enthusiasm
- love and strong relationships with family, friends, and colleagues.

Optimism is particularly relevant. The pessimist is fine until failure or setbacks occur. Then they catastrophize and fall apart. They think, "I'm a loser! I'll lose my job! Nobody loves me." The optimist says, "Well, here's the lesson. Here's how I can do better."

A big thing that separates happy from unhappy people is how they deal with setbacks. Optimism is a wonderful tool to have when setbacks occur.

For example, one thing I've learned for myself is that when a setback occurs, you should just take a deep breath and not do anything to make it worse. I get most of my bad news over e-mail. I've learned to never, never respond to an upsetting e-mail until the next day. Then it never seems as bad as when I first read it.

Another thing that's affected my own life as a result of our research is I now try to be much kinder to other people by being curious about their well-being. I take the time to ask how they're doing, to actually mean it, and really listen to what they say. It's not just for the sake of the other person, it's also for my own sake. It absolutely makes me feel better. I am happier in that moment and over the long term as I do it over and over.

The most important thing we've learned in recent years about happiness is that *people can do things to be happy.* People have always hoped this was true, but we now have good research that proves these simple strategies work:

TOP 3 PROVEN HAPPINESS-BUILDING STRATEGIES
- being grateful
- doing acts of kindness
- learning to savor things

(continued)

In my own life, I am more grateful now. Instead of just taking an inventory of things that are messed up, I stop and say, "Here are the things that are going well in my life."

I also try to savor the good things much more. I used to have a tendency to gobble my food. That's fine when it's terrible food. But a really good meal? You should chew every bite and savor it all the more.

An interesting question is when something pleasant or pleasurable happens, what do you do with it? Some people know how to prolong it, to get as much bang out of it as possible. I read an excellent book called *Savoring*, by Fred Bryant and Joseph Veroff, and I found some of their ideas very helpful.

For example, when something good happens, focus on it fully, and don't try to multitask! Let's say you get a nice letter from a loved one. Don't try to read the letter while you're watching TV or eating or flipping through your bills. Turn off the TV, sit down, read the letter slowly, maybe read it out loud. That's savoring. It has so much more of an impact.

I think all these things add up and multiply. I don't want to say I'm walking on sunshine, but they do have a cumulative effect. I certainly am happier now than I was twenty years ago. ∽

Happiness Breakthrough #6:
The Upward Spiral
of Positive Emotions

Life can present you with some very dark moments. And I've had my share.

I've gotten sick. I've had business setbacks. I've gotten divorced. I've had friends die tragically before their time. I've made all kinds of mistakes.

I'm a Type A personality, and when I wake up every morning I'm always looking for that next accomplishment. I put a lot of stress on myself to make things happen today, not three months from now. But daily life throws me curveballs and hand grenades. Things go wrong.

All of these, the big crises and the little nuisances, can push me into downward spirals of negative thinking and negative self-talk. I can get so caught up and bogged down in these negative downward spirals that it can feel like a free fall into despair. One morning last year I was feeling both lousy from my MS symptoms and stressed out by life, and I wound up standing in the shower crying, temporarily drowning in a flood of negative thoughts.

I started wondering if that grade school teacher was right—I'll never amount to anything! It's crazy, but no matter what the accomplishment, I often don't feel like I've ever achieved anything. I should be really proud that I got my show on national television and kept it there for thirty-two hundred episodes and seventeen years. But then a voice in the back of my brain says, "Hey, loser, why couldn't you keep it on the air for twenty years?"

I think all of us experience feelings of self-doubt, social anxiety, and negative self-talk. You can start thinking these insidious, self-undermining thoughts, which compound and feed on each other, like:

"You're not good enough for that job!"

"They'll ask you a question you won't know the answer to!"

"You'll start sweating!"

"Everyone will think you're a jerk!"

"They'll find out what a dummy you are!"

"They'll realize you're a fraud!"

"Your pants are going to split in the middle of the meeting!"

"Everything's going to go wrong today. I can feel it!"

We all think this way sometimes; it's just human nature. But with depressed people, these thoughts can become immobilizing, and they can fall into a crevasse of very dark thoughts, what one eminent psychiatrist called the "cognitive triad" of depression:

- "I'm no good.
- "My world is bleak.
- "My future is hopeless."

It is a vicious, self-sustaining cycle. "Rumination," noted Susan Nolen-Hoeksema, a professor of psychology at Yale University, "whether re-hashing things from the past or worrying about the future, worsens and lengthens periods of depression and can make everyday bad moods more intense."

Before I learned to manage my depression effectively, I would stay focused on thoughts like these and not know how to dig my way out of the emotional hole I'd fallen into. It felt like the walls were caving in.

It's weird, but certain behaviors can keep you focused on depression. Sometimes, just dealing with insensitive or sourpuss doctors made me feel codependent with them in my own depression. Other times, I think I wore my depression as a perverse kind of badge of courage, to prove to myself and the world how courageous and tough and interesting I am. I got caught up in the drama of being depressed. I've known people who have been stuck in old-fashioned Freudian-style therapy for ten years, focusing on childhood events and never really getting anywhere. I think it can be a waste of time to wallow in the past.

Whether you're depressed or just having a bad day, negative self-talk can really short-circuit your emotional life, there's no doubt about it.

One way of addressing this problem is with cognitive therapy, where a trained therapist helps you navigate your way into more productive and more fulfilling ways of thinking.

And I have discovered a truly amazing insight in my own life that is now being explored and increasingly understood by experts:

Just as there is a downward spiral of negative emotions, there is an upward spiral of positive emotions that build on each other to help you grow and thrive.

As it is in physics, where every action has an equal and opposite reaction, so it can be with our emotional lives.

When my emotional elevator starts to plunge into negativity, I make a strong, conscious effort to stop and ignite an upward spiral. I'll look for a sparkle of light to hold on to in the form of a positive thought, then another, then another. I do it almost every day. The positive thoughts will build on each other and lift me out of the plunge. And I believe you can ignite your own fire of your positive emotions in much the same way.

Barbara L. Fredrickson, a psychology professor at the University of North Carolina, has been studying this phenomenon intensely. After years of research and experimentation, she's come up with what she calls the "broaden and build" theory of positive emotions, a concept for which she won the Templeton Positive Psychology Prize.

Negative emotions, her theory goes, have a crucial evolutionary role. Our ancestors, for example, used the negative emotion of anger to defend the tribe and attack predators, and they used fear to escape danger. These emotions force human thinking to quicken and narrow down to only those actions needed for survival.

But positive emotions like joy, interest, serenity, gratitude, love, and contentment, according to Fredrickson, not only "broaden and build" on each other, they can "undo" or at least "loosen the hold" that negative emotions have on our mind and body, and spark what she calls a "mutually reinforcing ascent to greater well-being":

> ⤳ *Cultivating positive emotions produces an upward spiral that broadens habitual modes of thinking and acting, and builds personal resources for coping.*
>
> ⤳ *Over time, the broadening sparked by positive emotions creates an upward spiral that builds personal strength, resilience, and well-being.*
>
> —BARBARA L. FREDRICKSON

Four Tips to Trigger the
Upward Spiral of Positive Emotions

How can we trigger the upward spiral in our lives? One mega-strategy Professor Fredrickson has outlined is to *find positive meaning in our daily lives*. We can:

- Find positive meaning in adversity.
- Find positive meaning in ordinary events.
- Find positive meaning in compassionately helping others.
- Find positive meaning by feeling gratitude for simple things.

That, in my book, is a great formula for achieving happiness!

Happiness Breakthrough #7:
The Flow of Happiness

When have you been the most happy in your life?

Some of my absolute happiest times have been when my skills have been put to the test, I've faced a series of great challenges, and I plunged into them with all my heart and soul. I became so totally absorbed in the challenge that time seemed to stop and I entered a zone of pure energy, thought, and motion, all of which I controlled.

Right now, for example, I'm flying all around the country having meetings and doing deals for new TV and business ventures. I walk in the door supremely confident that no one can stop me. I'm not afraid of fumbling and I'm not afraid of failure. I wake up every morning, look at my mug in the mirror, and say to myself, "Today I'm going to set the world on fire." And I mean it!

It's the ultimate feeling of being "in the zone."

This feeling of total absorption is experienced every day by people

whose skills and challenges are matched and pushed into intense, productive action. It could be a construction worker who is great at her job, or
a musician who becomes "one with the music," or an accountant with a
talent and passion for balance sheets. It happens to new mothers who
spend their day caring for their newborns, when time melts away and all
that matters is the dance of intense connection between parent and child.

What we choose to do with our days, and how intensely we enjoy it,
has for ages been seen as a pathway to happiness, by philosophers, po-
ets, and athletes alike:

> *The happiness of a man is to do the true work of a man.*
>
> —MARCUS AURELIUS

> *The chiefest point of happiness is that a man should be willing
> to be what he is.*
>
> —ERASMUS

> *It is neither wealth, nor splendor, but tranquility and occupa-
> tion, which give happiness.*
>
> —THOMAS JEFFERSON

> *The only happiness a brave man ever troubled himself with ask-
> ing much about was, happiness enough to get his work done.*
>
> —THOMAS CARLYLE

> *A good life is one that is characterized by complete absorption
> in what one does.*
>
> —PROFESSOR JEANNE NAKAMURA

> *If you mess up, there's a good chance you could die. I'm just
> there, totally in the moment, in a heightened state of existence.*
>
> —JEFF MEYER, PROFESSIONAL SNOWBOARDER

You're going all out. By the end you can't walk, you can't see straight, you count down every second. Everything hurts. But sometimes, it just clicks. Time almost doesn't exist. There's a oneness, a wholeness. You're going on instinct; you just let your body take over.

—ERIN MIRABELLA, OLYMPIC TRACK CYCLIST

It almost feels like I'm running downhill. It's this feeling of total integration with your surroundings, everything being in its right place, a harmonious way of being. . . . It's about as spiritual and religious as I get.

—ANTON KRUPICKA, ULTRA RUNNER

You lose your sense of time, you're completely enraptured, and you're sort of swayed by the possibilities you see in this work. The idea is to be so saturated with it that there's no future or past, it's just an extended present in which you're making meaning.

—MARK STRAND, POET

There's one man who has studied the connections between complete absorption and happiness more than anyone else, and his name is Mihaly Csikszentmihalyi (pronounced "cheek-sent-me-high").

Over fifty years ago, the Hungarian-born Csikszentmihalyi decided to spend his life studying what made people happy.

He studied over ten thousand people, devoted thirty years and eighteen books to the subject, and came up with the simple word "flow" to describe the idea of intense concentration, the sensation he compares to "being carried away by an effortless current." The reason it enables happiness, he found, "is that it involves a challenge that matches one's ability."

The pathway to achieving lasting happiness, Professor Csikszentmihalyi concluded, is "to keep finding new opportunities to refine one's skills: do one's job better or faster, or expand the tasks that comprise it; find a new set of challenges more appropriate to your stage of life." He described the "flow experience" as stepping into a kind of parallel reality where you "forget the problems of everyday life." Ironically, it is only after the flow experience that happiness is fully enjoyed—not during it.

The formula for a flow experience, observed Csikszentmihalyi, is to have clear goals, immediate feedback on your performance, and a good balance between your skills and the challenge at hand.

> ᴂ In many ways, the secret to happiness is to learn to get flow from almost everything we do, including work and family commitments. If everything is worth doing for its own sake, then there is nothing wasted in life. The link between flow and happiness depends on whether the flow-producing activity is complex, whether it leads to new challenges and hence to personal and cultural growth.
>
> —PROFESSOR MIHALY CSIKSZENTMIHALYI

LIVING WELL EMOTIONALLY EXPERT
Professor Mihaly Csikszentmihalyi

Professor Mihaly Csikszentmihalyi is C. S. and D. J. Davidson Professor of Psychology and Management and director of the Quality of Life Research Center, or QLRC, at the Drucker School, the Claremont School of Management.

He is credited with being the cofounder, along with Professor Mar-

(continued)

tin Seligman, of the positive psychology movement. He is also considered the world's leading authority on the connections between "flow," or intense absorption, and happiness.

Professor Csikszentmihalyi is the author of Flow: The Psychology of Optimal Experience *and* Finding Flow: The Psychology of Engagement with Everyday Life.

The feeling of "flow" has the effect of creating a world, a paramount reality that is in a sense parallel to the one you live in.

It is the feeling of being able to control or master life, at least temporarily.

Where your flow comes from can change as you grow, and as you mature.

I remember being a boy in Hungary during World War II. These were very dark days, people were being killed and bombs were exploding. You never knew when you went to sleep at night what would happen to you. Those nights were when I started playing chess. I got immersed in the game, I felt completely in control of what I was doing. I forgot about everything else, I forgot the dangers and the misery of life.

In graduate school, I got a lot of flow from climbing mountains and doing rock climbing. Then I discovered painting, and it was the same feeling. You face a blank canvas and you put on a touch of color here and a line there and pretty soon you're living in a world you are actually making happen. It completely absorbs all of your attention.

Then I started enjoying writing. I wrote short stories, and a couple of them were published in the *New Yorker*. I was a correspondent for the French newspaper *Le Monde*. The writing was very absorbing. When you construct a story, whether it's fiction or nonfiction, you are in a sense creating a world of your own that you are making happen. Every move you make changes the story so it's kind of like painting or rock climbing.

More and more now, my flow comes from my work, and from relationships with friends and family. Relationships are highly creative: you have to make them grow, just like a story.

How can you apply flow in your life?

You have to make it happen. You have to choose something to do that you feel is worth investing your attention in, that you find interesting, that you are curious about. But it should also be something in which you will be able to grow, in which you can develop skills that will make you more and more able to interact with a new particular world, the world of new adventures you are developing.

Think about things you liked to do as a child or teenager, or something that you've never done because you didn't have the opportunity. Maybe you should try them now!

You can keep a "flow diary," where you write down what you really enjoy doing during each day, and write down what you didn't like doing each day. Keep it up for a couple of weeks, then look it over. Ask yourself, "Why am I doing these things I don't like to do? Can I get rid of some of those things, or figure out how to like them more? How can I do more of the things I actually do like?"

It's amazing, because people don't actually know this about themselves. Until they are really paying attention to it, they don't realize they could actually do more of what they love to do, as opposed to simply being glad when they happen. They could actually make them happen more often. It's very rare that people take charge of their own state of mind by saying, "I'm going to be more proactive and strategic about how I live—by trying to get the most out of life." ᓍ

CHAPTER 4

A Journey of the Body

This morning I went to the gym, did forty minutes of resistance training, got home and chugged a green smoothie for break-fast.

I was so pumped with energy that I was talking to myself in the shower, charging myself up for the day with positive self-talk: "Move it, Montel, come on, let's *go*! Get out there and conquer the world!"

Exercise makes me happy!

Nearly every single morning of my life, no matter where I am and how I'm feeling, I hit the gym first thing and work out for a full hour or hour and a half, rotating through the week the big three categories of exercise: aerobic-cardiovascular, resistance-strength, and flexibility-stretching.

I don't care where I am; if it's the pokiest hotel in nowhere land, there's a gym in there somewhere and I'll find it. If it's closed, I'll beg the manager into giving up the key.

I've been on one hell of a physical journey with multiple sclerosis. There are days when I can barely stand up and walk due to severe cramping, pain, and stiffness in my joints, and other days when I can't walk across the room without tripping.

But the daily ritual of exercise gives me a sense of achievement and control over my destiny, a sensation of power and strength, and feelings of peace, contentment, and physical joy, feelings that carry over directly into my mental and spiritual lives. Exercise gives me tremendous emotional benefits. It's a positive ritual, an affirmation, and something good I'm doing for myself that will help me live a better life.

All right, I'll admit it—exercise makes me a little high!

If exercise was a drug, and the results it delivered were available in a pill, it would be a hundred times hotter than Viagra. But tragically, more than 60 percent of American adults are not getting enough physical activity to achieve health benefits.

If you're not doing this drug most days of the week, believe me, it's time you got started. And getting happier is just one of the many reasons.

Why Exercise Is a Magic Bullet of Happiness

Here are just a few of the possible benefits associated with regular physical activity:

- Elevates mood and fights depression.
- Gives you more energy, enhances self-esteem, reduces feelings of stress and anxiety, helps you relax, and helps you sleep better.
- Increases the number of calories your body uses and helps you achieve a healthy body weight.
- Tones your body and strengthens your bones and muscles.
- Improves your stamina and overall fitness.
- Lowers your risk of heart disease, high blood pressure, obesity, metabolic syndrome, type 2 diabetes, Alzheimer's disease, osteoarthritis, osteoporosis, and erectile dysfunction.
- Reduces your number of hospitalizations, physician visits, and medications.
- Increases your odds of looking and feeling healthy, sexy, and fabulous.

For people like me with a chronic disease, exercise is especially important for strengthening the body in the face of the disease's physical assaults. Multiple sclerosis, for example, produces fatigue, poor balance, weakness, spasticity, heat sensitivity, and mental depression. On top of that, MS symptoms can cause physical inactivity, which can in turn develop into new, debilitating secondary diseases. The good news is that, in the words of one team of researchers, "a growing number of studies indicate that exercise in patients with mild-to-moderate MS provides similar fitness and psychological benefits" as it does with healthy people.

I believe your physical well-being is directly and powerfully interconnected with your mental state and your moods. Having your mind healthy helps your physical well-being, and vice versa. They are totally intertwined. The exercise you do and the food you eat can have as much of an impact on your emotional well-being as any pill you can take.

You may think I'm an exercise nut, and you'd be right if you did. But the idea of exercise as a mood booster is increasingly popular among doctors and scientists, too:

> *Exercise is the first step for all my patients. It boosts everyone.*
>
> —Dr. Richard A. Friedman,
> Psychologist and Director of Pharmacology,
> Payne Whitney Institute, Cornell
> Presbyterian Medical Center

> *I can't overstate how important regular exercise is in improving the function and performance of the brain. It's such a wonderful medicine. Exercise is as good as any antidepressant I know.*
>
> —Dr. John Ratey,
> Associate Professor of Psychiatry,
> Harvard Medical School

A brisk five-to-ten-minute walk is all you need to get a mood benefit. No sweat required.

— PROFESSOR ROBERT THAYER,
PROFESSOR OF PSYCHOLOGY,
CALIFORNIA STATE UNIVERSITY

Our results suggest that more physical activity is associated with reduced concurrent depression. In addition, it appears that physical activity may be especially helpful in the context of medical problems and major life stressors. Clinically, encouraging depressed patients to engage in physical activity is likely to have potential benefits with few obvious risks.

— ALEXANDER HARRIS AND COLLEAGUES,
AUTHORS OF A VETERANS ADMINISTRATION–STANFORD UNIVERSITY
MEDICAL SCHOOL TEN-YEAR STUDY OF PHYSICAL ACTIVITY

Scientists have long suspected that exercise can boost your mood, making you happier and less depressed. Many research studies suggested the connection existed, but the studies were usually small, of brief duration, and did not compare exercise versus a placebo. That changed in 2007 when a major study was published by a team of researchers led by Professor James A. Blumenthal, a professor of medical psychology at Duke University Medical Center in Durham, North Carolina.

Professor Blumenthal's team assigned 202 men and women age forty and older who were diagnosed with major depression to one of four treatments: a supervised exercise program; a home-based aerobic exercise program; the antidepressant sertraline (Zoloft); and placebo pills. After sixteen weeks, the patients in the supervised exercise group improved at almost the same rate as those taking the antidepressant. And six months later, patients who exercised had half the risk of being depressed as those who didn't.

This is terrific news. The effectiveness of exercise, the researchers found, "seems generally comparable with patients receiving antidepressant medication and both tend to be better than the placebo in patients with MDD [major depressive disorder]. Placebo response rates were high, suggesting that a considerable portion of the therapeutic response is determined by patient expectations, ongoing symptom monitoring, attention, and other nonspecific factors."

One limitation of the study was that it did not look at the effects of psychotherapy, and another is that the patients studied were receptive to the idea of exercising. Dr. Blumenthal concluded, "There is certainly growing evidence that exercise may be a viable alternative to medication, at least among those patients who are receptive to exercise as a potential treatment for their depression."

It's only recently that experts have figured out how beneficial physical activity is. By the way, I'm using the terms "exercise" and "physical activity" fairly interchangeably, since I see them as part of the same continuum. Physical activity can be highly structured exercise or "incidental exercise" that comes from an active lifestyle. It all counts and it all adds up, as long as you're moving!

Exactly how does exercise make us happy? Scientists still aren't sure. So far they don't have much evidence, but they have plenty of hypotheses.

The "brain theories" speculate that a rise in temperature following exercise affects sections of the brain that reduce muscular tension and creates feelings of relaxation; exercise boosts the availability of brain neurotransmitters like serotonin and dopamine that are reduced with depression; or that exercise protects and improves brain health. The "self-efficacy theory" maintains that exercise strengthens the belief that one has the skills to achieve an objective, and the confidence to complete the task, both of which can increase positive thinking and reduce depressive feelings. The "distraction theory" holds that physical activity helps distract us from negative and depressing thoughts.

Personally, I'd bet that they're all true. We've all heard of endorphins and runner's high creating bursts of happiness or euphoria. For more than thirty years, experts believed that exercise released a flood of endorphins, or natural opiate-like hormones, in the brain, but they couldn't really prove it.

Then last year, a team of researchers at the University of Bonn reported using advances in neuro-scanning technology to measure runners after they ran for two hours, and sure enough, they discovered that after exercise, endorphins really were active in the brain. The positive mood, calmness, euphoria of "runner's high" is not a myth, but a flesh-and-blood happiness by-product of exercise.

I totally buy into the endorphin theory. I believe it and I live it. Practically every day, after I've done a session of aerobic training on the elliptical machine, I absolutely feel a simultaneous burst of energy and peace in my brain.

I can't really flat out run anymore, and I don't think it would be a pretty sight, to be honest with you—lots of tripping and face-planting. But for those who can run, it may deliver especially powerful anti-depression benefits. An article published in a respected medical journal, the *Journal of Clinical Psychiatry*, reported that "running has been compared with psychotherapy in the treatment of depression, with results indicating that running is just as effective as psychotherapy in alleviating symptoms of depression."

Another excellent potential ticket to happiness is walking—extra-cheap, super-easy, plain, old-fashioned walking.

Robert Thayer, a professor of psychology at California State University in Long Beach, has said that "the more a person walks has a very real and immediate psychological effect that an individual can experience every day." He and his students conducted a study of twelve males and twenty-five females who wore pedometers over a twenty-day period, and measured mood, self-esteem, happiness, depression, and energy and tension levels.

"We found that there was a clear and strong relationship between the number of steps they took and their overall mood and energy level," reported Professor Thayer, adding, "In this whole series of studies that we've done, the more you walk in a day, the more energy you experience." The effects were simple: when the subjects walked more, they rated more highly their health, energy, overall mood, happiness, and self-esteem.

In his book *Calm Energy*, Thayer identified a central paradox of the equation: the more depressed people are, the less they want to exercise. "Exercising would be the best thing for them, but they are too tired or too depressed to do it," he explained. "So, it is important to get the word out and make people realize that if they get up and walk or exercise, they will feel better."

There's another paradox at work here, though it's really more like an enormous human tragedy. Every year, hundreds of thousands of stressed-out, sad, or depressed people are marching into their primary care doctors or psychiatrists, and walking out with prescriptions for medicine, and hopefully for therapy, too, but not once does the word "exercise" pass the doctors' lips, or even enter the doctors' brains! Not once! How tragic is that?

That medicine may well be a lifesaver for those patients, but hey, come on; they're forgetting an entire piece of the equation!

You may say I'm a dreamer, but I want every psychiatrist's office in America to be equipped with a treadmill. When a patient comes in, the psychiatrist says, "Get on this machine and walk for twenty minutes while we talk. Let's go, baby—walk!" Now that would make sense! The right forms of exercise can be cheap, easy, and effective depression fighters and mood boosters.

Tips for Boosting Your Mood
Through Exercise

- If you're just beginning an exercise lifestyle, work with your doctor, and start slow.
- Set small, achievable goals: for example, three exercise sessions per week, at a comfortable pace, for ten minutes each. Then gradually increase the duration and intensity over time.
- If you think it would help, get your friends and family involved and make exercise a group or buddy challenge and activity.
- Monitor your progress with a pedometer or a simple exercise log, where you jot down your daily targets and progress.
- Keep an "Emotional Exercise Journal" in which you write down the positive feelings you experience after every time you exercise.
- Realize that physical activity does not have to be strenuous to be beneficial.
- "Exercise snacks" of short bursts of activity, at least ten minutes in duration—like short power walks, climbing stairs, gardening, and vacuuming—all count as physical activity.
- If you're depressed, realize that exercise may provide strong benefits for helping you feel better. But also recognize that depression may make it hard for you to muster the energy and motivation to exercise right away, that you should get professional help, and that medication and therapy can also be very effective in helping you feel better.
- In addition to the "big 3" traditional forms of exercise—aerobic, strength, and flexibility—you can explore new and alternative mind and body methods like yoga, tai chi, meditation, and relaxation techniques.

Your Living Well Emotionally Physical Activity Target

• Gradually begin working toward the target of at least thirty to sixty minutes of moderate physical activity, such as brisk walking, on most days of the week.

LIVING WELL EMOTIONALLY EXPERT
Professor James A. Blumenthal

James A. Blumenthal, Ph.D., is a Professor of Medical Psychology at Duke University Medical Center and Professor of Psychology in the Department of Psychology and Neurosciences.

He holds fellowship status in the American Psychological Association, the Society of Behavioral Medicine and the Academy of Behavioral Medicine Research and is a founding fellow of the American Association of Cardiovascular and Pulmonary Rehabilitation. He also has served as president of the American Psychosomatic Society and is a former president of Division 38 (Health) of the American Psychological Association.

His research focuses on psychosocial factors and health and behavioral interventions in primary and secondary prevention of cardiovascular and pulmonary disease.

Professor Blumenthal has directed a number of clinical trials in behavioral medicine, including the SMILE Study, which is the largest randomized trial to date that investigated the connections between exercise and mental health.

People who are more physically active are less likely to be depressed. The data are pretty consistent, and we see it in a number of different populations.

(continued)

We've also observed that nondepressed patients experience reductions in depressive symptoms when they exercise.

The question is, does depression cause people to be less active, or are people who are less active more likely to be depressed? It's a chicken-and-egg phenomenon and we really don't know the answer.

Some people consider an absence of depression to be happiness, whereas others believe that happiness represents its own independent but related concept. There have been fewer studies on the impact of exercise on happiness than on the reduction in depressive symptoms. But anecdotally, people report that they are happier when they exercise, they're functioning better, and they're enjoying life more.

The first study that we did in 1999, which was published in the *Archives of Internal Medicine*, and a follow-up study published in *Psychosomatic Medicine* compared exercise, antidepressants, and a combination of the two. The result was, first and most important, that everybody got better.

Second, even the patients with more severe depression benefited from the exercise alone. That was a bit of a surprise for us.

When we followed up with them six months after they completed the program, we found that patients who had been in the exercise group were much less likely to have relapsed. Their relapse rate was 9 percent compared to over 30 percent in the groups that got medication.

Why is exercise having this effect? There's a lot we don't yet know about brain biochemistry. It may be a psychological mechanism that trickles down to the brain chemistry, where people who exercise feel more of a sense of accomplishment, more hopeful, more in control.

I know I feel better when I'm more physically active, when I exercise regularly. I try to exercise at least five days a week, if not every day. Today I will go out on my bike for an hour. I try to build some kind of physical activity into every day.

What is the optimal dose of exercise for reducing depressive symptoms? We found that three days a week was adequate to provide benefits. Obviously, the biggest hurdle is going from doing no exercise to doing any exercise. Just take that first step and begin a program.

Of course there are certain days when you just don't have the time; as long as you recognize it's temporary and you'll get back to the routine, that's okay. But if you fall into a pattern where you can't find any time to exercise, then you need to adjust your lifestyle. You should reprioritize.

There are a lot of skeptics. There are physicians who would much rather write a prescription for a pill than for exercise, because that's what they do: you go to Midas, you get a muffler; you see a doctor, you get a prescription. That may be part of it. Or they may be unaware of the evidence for the benefits of exercise, or see flaws in the evidence.

If you're depressed, the biggest hurdle to exercising is simply getting over the inertia caused by depression. And if you're thinking you have to exercise heavily for the rest of your life, it could feel overwhelming and you'd never get started. But you don't have to be an Ironman triathlete. Exercise doesn't have to be highly intensive to be effective.

Here's an easy way to get started: decide that you're going to take a brisk walk three times a week for twenty minutes each. That would definitely be a good start, and I'd be very optimistic that that would result in benefits for you. Charting your progress can help—put a little calendar on your refrigerator and jot down your achievement each day. Keep in mind the benefits: you'll lose weight, you'll have more energy, and you'll feel better.

Just try it for a short period of time and see how you do. Just *try* it! ✑

LIVING WELL EMOTIONALLY EXPERT
Dr. John Ratey

John J. Ratey, M.D., is an Associate Clinical Professor of Psychiatry at Harvard Medical School.

As a clinical researcher he has published more than sixty papers in peer-review journals in the fields of psychiatry and psychopharmacology.

For more than a decade he taught residents and Harvard medical students as the Assistant Director of Resident Training at Massachusetts Mental Health Center. He continues to teach psychiatrists as a regular instructor in Harvard's Continuing Medical Education program.

In 1986 he founded the Boston Center for the Study of Autism, and in 1988 he founded a new study group of the American Psychiatric Association focused on the study of aggression, which grew out of his research and development of novel drug treatments for aggressive behavior. During this time he lectured internationally on aggression and disturbances in the brain that affect social functioning.

Dr. Ratey began studying ADHD in the 1980s and coauthored Driven to Distraction: Recognizing and Coping with Attention Deficit Disorder from Childhood through Adulthood, *the first in a series of books that demystify the disorder. He also coauthored* Shadow Syndromes *with Catherine Johnson, Ph.D., in which he describes the phenomenon of milder forms of clinical disorders. His latest book is* Spark: The Revolutionary New Science of Exercise and the Brain.

Since 1998 Dr. Ratey has been selected each year as one of the best doctors in America by his peers. He was the recipient of the 2006 Excellence in Advocacy Award from the nonprofit group PE4Life, for his work to promote the adoption of regular, aerobic-based physical education.

What I know is that when I exercise it gives me a feeling of energy and interest, and my motivation and vigor go up. Every morning, the first thing in the morning, I stop at the gym.

One advantage exercise has over antidepressants is the feeling of self-efficacy. You are getting out there and pushing yourself. You are the agent of change, not a pill. It's a very positive feeling.

Exercise has such a big effect on the brain. It can help depression, stress, anxiety, attention deficit disorder, and mood regulation. Recent studies looked at students in inner-city schools who were moved from once-a-week exercise to daily exercise of thirty to forty-five minutes. The results were very compelling. The first effect was a drop in aggression and anger. Within just three months there was a 50 percent drop in disciplinary referrals and an even higher drop in days of suspension. There were also improvements in focus, attention, and motivation.

It's a crime that our culture has become so sedentary. Many of the diseases we have today could be reduced by an active lifestyle: cardiac problems, diabetes and arthritis, certain kinds of cancer. Take Alzheimer's, for example. With an active lifestyle you can reduce your risk of getting Alzheimer's by 50 percent.

If you're sedentary, just start moving and walking. Make it a part of your life. Get a pedometer and a cardiac monitor to determine what your fitness zones are. The more you walk, the better you'll feel. You should be walking at least forty minutes, six days a week. Some of those days, you should really push it by either walking uphill or extra briskly. Get to the point where you're increasing the challenges you take on.

Set aside some time every day, or almost every day, for exercise. Make

(continued)

a commitment with a friend to help each other. Get outside and exercise in nature, fresh air, and sunshine.

Weight training should be a part of everybody's routine. Everybody over forty should also do strength training and some balance work.

How does exercise promote happiness?

We believe it elevates neurotransmitters like serotonin and dopamine, and also promotes neuroplasticity of the brain, which helps the brain change and adapt. Depression may be in part a shutdown of neuroplasticity. Improved neuroplasticity in your brain may help reverse "learned helplessness," or feelings like "there's nothing out there for me, so why bother." Part of happiness is feeling that the world is full of possibilities. With exercise, you get a snap-back and reemergence of neuroplasticity. Exercise does this as effectively as anything we know.

Exercise also promotes two more antidepressant factors in your body. The first is called BDNF-1, or what I call "Miracle-Gro for the brain." It is involved in mood, in learning, in feeling optimistic. The second factor is endocannabanoids, which I call our body and brain's "internal marijuana," or THC, which promotes feelings of well-being. Exercise really jumps them up. ☙

LIVING WELL EMOTIONALLY EXPERT
Professor Robert Thayer

Robert E. Thayer, Ph.D., is Professor of Psychology at California State University, Long Beach, where he teaches "The Psychology of Mood" and other courses.

He is the author of The Biopsychology of Mood and Arousal, The Origin of Everyday Moods, *and* Calm Energy: How People Regulate Mood with Food and Exercise. *His work is widely cited in the scientific literature and the press.*

He is a leading researcher on the connections between physical activity, mood, and happiness.

I call the state of high energy and low tension "calm energy."

Calm energy and happiness line up closely together. One of the ways to achieve calm energy is by exercise, such as brisk walking at a rate of about four miles an hour.

Walking is an immediate pathway to a form of happiness. We are seeing research that moderate depression is strongly affected by exercise, and even serious forms of depression are probably affected by exercise.

In our research, we had people wear pedometers for three weeks and compare the days they walked more to the days they walked less. It was very clear that on the days they walked more they were happier, and on the days they walked less, they were less happy.

It's amazing how long the energy effect lasts. One study found that after a ten-minute walk, the effect of increased energy lasted up to two hours.

How does this happen? I call it general bodily arousal. If you're sitting quietly in a baseline condition, various systems of the body are at rest.

(continued)

When you get up and begin to walk, your body is activated at all levels: increased metabolism and cardiovascular activity; increased endocrines like cortisol and adrenaline; and greater volume of neurotransmitters and neuromodulators in certain parts of the brain, like dopamine, serotonin, and norepinephrine. They are all integrated with each other. The way you know they're activated is through the feeling of increased energy you feel.

When you walk more, you have increased energy. It's a very significant effect. Happiness is probably driven by energy, and when you feel more energy, you feel happier.

When we did a research study with depressed women, we found that they were significantly less depressed and more energetic on the days they walked fifteen minutes than on the days they didn't. But some of the women in the group we started with were just too depressed to walk. It's a real problem; when you're depressed your energy drops, and you can feel too tired to walk or exercise. My advice is to try what I call a "cognitive override," where you overrule the negative impulses to stay sedentary—by remembering how much better the exercise is going to make you feel.

You would think that on the basis of what we know, exercise should be the Holy Grail of our society. Everybody agrees on how important it is. You'd think people would be exercising more and more. But people are exercising less and less, because they're working more and feel they don't have time to work out.

Ironically, I think they would be much more productive and effective at their work if they exercised more, because of the positive mood and happiness they would experience!

Just try it. You can try it in relatively small amounts.

Don't think you've got to go to a gym and work out for an hour at first. If you're just getting started, just get up and walk fifty steps, or get out and walk down the street. You'll feel different—you'll feel better. As soon as you begin to do that, your system becomes activated, your body aroused, and you'll feel the benefit right away.

You should also know that your energy will vary throughout the day, in a circadian rhythm, in what I call an endogenous biological rhythm. It's like a built-in clock, and the pattern is the same day after day. You start out with low energy when you first wake up in the morning. Then for most people your energy ramps up to the highest point in late morning or early afternoon, then it drops off in the late afternoon. There's a subpeak in the early evening, then your energy drops to the lowest point just before you go to sleep.

This energy cycle often affects the degree to which you are influenced by stress and anxiety. When energy is low, you are much more vulnerable to tension and anxiety, and the world can look dark and problematic.

Studies show that the same problem can look more serious at different times of day, depending on this energy and tension variation. Late in the afternoon or late at night, people tend to struggle with their lives and focus on how terrible things are, but the next morning when experiencing more energy and less tension, problems look less serious.

You should remember that your mood and your emotional feelings can be influenced by something as simple as what time of day it is. ⟨⟨

CATCH SOME RAYS:
THE PROMISE OF LIGHT THERAPY

The other day I got the urge to soak my face in sunlight.

It was a beautiful clear day, so I sat down on a park bench, closed my eyes, and luxuriated in pure sun juice. Time melted away, stress disappeared, and all I heard was the chirping of birds and the laughter of children echoing over the hills of Central Park. If I'd planned ahead I would have brought some sunscreen, but what the heck.

By the end of those twenty minutes I might have been the happiest guy on Planet Earth. It was like a feast of happy feelings and emotions: peace, contentment, serenity, joy, euphoria. My body and mind were high on sun.

If you suffer from depression, the power of light is a fascinating pathway to potentially improving your mood. "Light therapy," an experimental treatment using a light box (which can cost $200 to $400) that filters out harmful ultraviolet rays, and "dawn simulation," a variation of the treatment that simulates the time and strength of a normal daily sunrise, have shown great promise in helping depressed people feel better.

For more than twenty-five years, experts have been studying bright light exposure as a treatment for one form of depression called seasonal affective disorder (SAD). SAD is not considered a unique mood disorder, but as an indication of major depression that tends to recur at specific times of the year, especially winter, when sunlight is reduced. Symptoms can include social withdrawal, fatigue, food cravings, and sleep disruption.

Recently, scientists have been extending their studies of light therapy beyond SAD to see if it can help conditions like non-seasonal major depressive disorder and bipolar depression, postpartum depression, and adult attention deficit hyperactivity disorder.

So far, the research on light therapy has been limited, but very promising.

A major review published in the *American Journal of Psychiatry* in 2005 about light therapy and mood disorders found that "randomized, controlled trials suggest that bright light treatment and dawn simulation for seasonal affective disorder and bright light for non-seasonal depression are efficacious, with effect sizes equivalent to those in most antidepressant pharmacotherapy trials." When the authors of the review analyzed the data they found "significant reduction in depression symptom severity following bright light therapy in seasonal affective disorder and in non-seasonal depression, as well as a significant effect with dawn simulation in seasonal affective disorder."

Much research remains to be done. It's not yet known if light therapy is as effective as drug therapy, and how it interacts with or complements either talk therapies or medications.

Experts don't know what the ideal dose is. Treatment times can vary from fifteen to ninety minutes a day, in various weekly schedules, and various intensities from 2,500 lux ("lux" is a measure of light strength) per session to 10,500 lux. Light therapy is thought to be more effective earlier in the day. Some possible side effects have been reported, including headache, eyestrain, nausea, and irritability.

If you suffer from depression, you should check with your doctor to see if light therapy would be a promising treatment for you.

CHAPTER 5

The Happiness Diet

One vision of happiness is to see it as living a healthy life, with the lowest risk of chronic diseases.

I can think of few feelings as happy as enjoying beautiful health and positive physical energy, and few situations as sad or depressing as getting heart disease, or cancer, or going blind, or having limbs amputated as a result of type 2 diabetes.

As a nation, we are overwhelmed: with excessive sugar, especially from useless sugary soft drinks; with excessive sodium; with excessive consumption of junk food like candy and potato chips; with too much heart-unhealthy saturated fat; and way too much overprocessed food saturated in chemicals. At the same time, we are woefully undernourished in nutrients from fruits, vegetables, and whole grains; and omega-3 fatty acids from foods like fish.

The result: hundreds of thousands of Americans are suffering today from a raging epidemic of diseases that were largely triggered by bad diet and physical inactivity. It's no secret that the typical American diet and couch-potato lifestyle are a disaster, a slow-motion horror movie that is literally killing hundreds of thousands of people before their time.

But here's the great news.

There is a dietary and lifestyle pattern that is emerging as a consensus recommendation among many health authorities and experts as a pattern that can reduce your risk of a wide range of major diseases, such as cardiovascular disease, obesity, several forms of cancer, type 2 diabetes, Alzheimer's disease, osteoarthritis, and macular degeneration, all of which can have a devastating effect on your well-being. It's a pattern I called "The Living Well Code" in my last book. It's also a pattern you can call "The Happiness Diet":

1. Base your diet on a foundation of a rich variety of many different vegetables and fruits—especially in their unprocessed states.

2. Include healthy carbohydrates from whole grains and healthy fats and protein from foods like fish, beans, and nuts.

3. Minimize saturated and trans fats, sodium, processed foods, added sugars, and cholesterol in your diet.

4. Be mindful of your calories-in and calories-out, to work toward a healthy body weight.

5. Don't skip meals, starve yourself, or go on fad diets.

6. Get regular physical activity: at least thirty to sixty minutes of moderate exercise on most days of the week.

That exceedingly simple formula, when put into action by you, is *one of the biggest keys to physical happiness and feeling fantastic you will ever find.*

It's only about a hundred words, but it synthesizes the wisdom of literally thousands of experts and scientific studies. There's a lot the experts don't know yet about what the perfect diet should look like, but the Happiness Diet comes close to their best judgment as of today.

A "plant-based diet," rich in vegetables, fruit, and whole grains, is emerging as the gold standard of nutrition. These are truly "happy foods."

Healthy carbohydrates like whole grains provide energy for our brains and bodies, and fiber for our digestive system.

Veggies and fruit are low in calorie density, or calories per bite, so they help us achieve a healthy body weight by filling us up on fewer calories. They contain multitudes of plant compounds and nutrients like vitamins, minerals, fiber, antioxidants, and phytochemicals, which appear to work together symphonically to fight many diseases and promote overall health.

Elite categories of extra-nutrient-rich veggies and fruits include leafy greens, cruciferous veggies like broccoli and cauliflower, sweet potatoes, berries, beans and nuts. The key is to eat lots of different kinds of produce.

Lowering our intake of saturated fat, trans fat, and sodium can deliver great benefits for our heart health. Being aware of our calorie intake and working toward a healthy body weight is seen by experts on heart disease, obesity, cancer, and other diseases as a key preventive step. And physical activity delivers a host of health benefits, and emotional benefits as well.

All these steps taken together can also reduce inflammation and boost our immune systems. "Inflammation appears to be a common thread of many chronic diseases of aging, like Alzheimer's, heart disease, diabetes, and common forms of cancer," said Dr. David Heber, director of the University of California, Los Angeles, Center for Human Nutrition.

The lesson of the Happiness Diet: Food is not your enemy. It's a pathway to joy and happiness.

Don't worry about "forbidden foods." For happiness, health, and living well, restrictive diets don't work over the long term. Positive thinking, flexible restraint, and allowing yourself treats and indulgences do.

Don't worry too much about what you *can't* have—focus on enjoying the multitudes of food you can enjoy. And enjoy indulgences—there's nothing intrinsically wrong with burgers, pizza, cookies, and chocolate—just make them occasional treats, not the focus of your diet. Rather than focusing on excluding anything from your diet, think about *adding in* healthy foods and working toward a healthy overall eating pattern.

THE HAPPY POWER OF FISH

There is one piece of the Happiness Diet that is especially exciting for improving our emotional health: fish and omega-3 fatty acids.

> ∽ *The data from randomized studies in major depression, suicide, and aggression indicate that fish is a food with psychotropic properties because it is rich in long chain omega-3 fatty acids that improve mental well-being, that is, change emotional states.*
>
> —Dr. Joseph Hibbeln

> ∽ *Many nutrition experts believe that humans once consumed omega-3 and omega-6 fatty acids in roughly equal amounts. But most North Americans and Europeans now get far too much of the omega-6s and not enough of the omega-3s. This dietary imbalance may explain the rise of such diseases as asthma, coronary heart disease, many forms of cancer, autoimmunity and neurodegenerative diseases, all believed to stem from inflammation in the body. The imbalance between*

omega-3 and omega-6 fatty acids may also contribute to obesity, depression, dyslexia, hyperactivity, and even a tendency toward violence.

—Dr. Andrew Weil

There is a scientist in Bethesda, Maryland, who thinks he has discovered a secret of happiness so powerful that it could change the world.

His name is Dr. Joseph Hibbeln. He is a commander in the United States Public Health Service, a medical doctor, and a biochemist. After twenty years of research, he believes that omega-3 fatty acids, found in fish and a few other foods, as well as fish oil supplements, have the potential to make us happier, make us less depressed, reduce stress, and help us in treating a variety of mental and emotional problems. On top of that, they can protect us against heart attacks.

What's more, Dr. Hibbeln is convinced that if populations could be persuaded to increase their consumption of omega-3 fatty acids, they would see a significant reduction in the rates of homicide, suicide, violence and aggressive behavior, feelings of despair, and personality disorders. The bulk of research so far on omega-3s and mental health has looked at reducing depression, not increasing happiness. But Hibbeln thinks that more happiness is where all this could lead.

If he is right, we could easily change the world for the better, and dramatically improve our own emotional well-being, simply by eating more fish or popping fish oil capsules.

Scientists had been intrigued by the potential benefits of omega-3 fatty acids from fish since the 1960s, when they noticed that Inuit populations who ate huge amounts of whale and seal blubber had very little heart disease.

They've noticed that Japan, too, consumes vast quantities of fish and experiences surprisingly low rates of sudden cardiac death, despite high rates of tobacco use and an increasingly unhealthy Westernized diet. Today, many experts and health authorities are urging us to eat more fish, as a strategy for protecting our hearts.

In the 1980s, Dr. Hibbeln started researching the possibility that omega-3s were also beneficial for our mental and emotional health. He noted that over the last century, the balance between omega-6 fatty acids and omega-3 fatty acids exploded from roughly 1 to 1 to a whopping 16 to 1 in favor of omega-6s, largely from industrial oils such as soya, corn, sunflower, and cottonseed used for industrial-scale frying and processing of foods. Since omega-6s reduce the brain-healthy effects of omega-3s, his theory went, the result was widespread mental and emotional problems.

His conclusions are not yet universally accepted, and there are limits to how far science can validate his theories. Hibbeln himself says that much more research is needed. But Dr. Hibbeln's observations and their implications are striking.

Studying thirty-six different nations, Hibbeln and his colleagues noticed striking possible connections between low fish consumption and high rates of various mental illnesses. Countries with the most rates of depression ate the least fish, and vice versa. Countries with the highest rates of fish consumption have lower rates of homicide, bipolar disorder, suicide, and seasonal affective disorder (SAD). The studies don't prove cause and effect, but they do point to possible connections.

One analysis reported that women who have more DHA (one of the omega-3 fatty acids) in their breast milk had lower rates of postpartum depression than women with less DHA. Another study found that omega-3 fatty acid supplementation could improve the response to existing antidepressant therapy.

There are plant sources of omega-3 fatty acid, too, like flaxseeds and walnuts. These are healthy foods, but Dr. Hibbeln doesn't believe they provide the same mood boost as fatty fish or fish oil capsules since the type of omega-3 in these sources isn't absorbed in the body as readily as the kind from fish.

Exactly how do omega-3s benefit our brain health and emotional health?

Experts aren't sure, but they have some good hypotheses. They may boost the levels of two neurotransmitters: serotonin, which is associated with reduced risk of depression, suicide, and violent behavior; and dopamine, which controls the brain's reward processes. They may improve blood flow to the brain. And they may protect brain cells and promote their growth.

Tips for Tapping the Happy Potential of Omega-3s and Fish

- What's the ideal dose of fish, or omega-3 supplements, to take? Scientists don't know yet. More may not necessarily be better. One possible side effect of omega-3 is its ability to thin blood, a special concern if you are taking daily aspirin or other blood thinners. Discuss with your doctor.
- Before changing your diet or taking any supplements, talk it over with your doctor.

Unfortunately, there are problems with some fish, in the form of mercury and other pollutants.

In 2004, the U.S. Environmental Protection Agency and the Food and Drug Administration issued an advisory that women should limit their fish consumption during pregnancy to 340 grams per week or less, due to concerns over potential neurotoxicity resulting from exposures to trace amounts of methylmercury.

Making things even more confusing, Dr. Hibbeln and his colleagues then published a response in the respected medical journal *The Lancet* that asserted that the net effect of limiting seafood consumption actually was "an increased risk of the detrimental effects the advisory intended to prevent." Specifically, the scientists concluded, there was a *greater* risk of children with lower verbal IQ and motor, communications, and social skills by age three when seafood consumption was limited.

The bottom line is that many fish are potentially polluted with trace amounts of methylmercury, and many others aren't.

There are, fortunately, good sources of fish information you can tap into on the Web, such as the excellent oceansalive.org Web site.

Oceansalive.org's "Good Fish"

These types of fish have three advantages: they're high in omega-3s, low in environmental contaminants, and harvested in an ecologically responsible manner:

- anchovies
- mackerel, Atlantic (not king mackerel, which can be high in toxic mercury)
- oysters (farmed)
- sablefish (Alaska, Canada)
- salmon (Alaska, canned)
- salmon, wild (Alaska)
- sardines, Pacific (U.S.)
- trout, rainbow (farmed)
- tuna, albacore (U.S., Canada)

LIVING WELL EMOTIONALLY EXPERT
Dr. Joseph Hibbeln

Dr. Joseph Hibbeln is the world's leading authority on an intriguing, crucial subject: the connections between omega-3 fatty acids and fish, and emotional well-being.

Dr. Hibbeln is a captain in the United States Public Health Service, a physician, a lipid biochemist, and an epidemiologist. He is Acting Chief, Section on Nutritional Neurochemistry of the Laboratory of Membrane Biophysics and Biochemistry, National Institute on Alcohol Abuse and Alcoholism at the National Institutes of Health.

Hibbeln was one of the first investigators to draw attention to the importance of omega-3 fatty acids in psychiatric disorders.

His work highlights the tremendous positive impact that omega-3 fatty acids, especially from fish, may have on our emotional health.

Our brains, our hearts, and our immune systems are absolutely dependent upon what we eat—and what dietary fats we eat.

There is very substantial evidence that omega-3 fatty acids treat depression as effectively or more effectively than do antidepressants, except they have no adverse side effects. They're cheaper, and they have secondary health benefits, such as protecting us from heart disease mortality.

Through the American Psychiatric Association, we have issued landmark treatment recommendations that unfortunately are little known to the public and the psychiatric community. They have just not been widely disseminated, due to a lack of promotional funds. The recommendations are for patients with most psychiatric illnesses to consume omega-3 fatty acids in the form of at least 1 gram of eicosapentaenoic acid (EPA) and docosa-

(continued)

hexaenoic acid (DHA) per day; or alternatively to eat three fish meals per week, especially fatty fish.

Over millions of years of human evolution, our diets were adapted to a diet that is very rich in fish. We evolved not on savannas, but on lakeshores and seashores. Hunting played some part, but it is thought by many physical anthropologists that the reason human beings were able to develop brains that are so large in proportion to the rest of our bodies is that we filled a dietary niche where we had abundant access to omega-3 fatty acids from fish.

But in the last hundred years in the U.S. we have been eating a diet with very little fish. And we've done something else. We've flooded our bodies and diets with a competing fatty acid called omega-6, from sources like corn oil and soybean oil, which drives down the beneficial effects of omega-3s.

Data we have on happiness and omega-3s come from a double-blind randomized placebo-controlled trial conducted upon people who presented to an emergency room for some episode of deliberate self-injury or self-harm. They were given either omega-3 fatty acids or a placebo.

There were several different findings: one is that they reduced their suicidal thinking by about a third. Next, they reduced their depression by about a half. And in the area of happiness, based on what's called the "Daily Hassles and Uplift Scale," those receiving omega-3 fatty acids reported about a one-third increase in positive perceptions of the little traumas of life. For example, you go to the airport and you're delayed by a security search. You can either perceive that as being a pain in the butt, or you can say, "Wow, this is great, I'm being so much better protected."

The bulk of the data that we have for omega-3s and emotions is in the reduction of depression, the reduction of anxiety, and the reduction of aggression.

For example, we've looked at thirty-six different countries, and the countries that eat more seafood per capita have lower homicide rates, lower bipolar depression, lower postnatal and other depression. These cross-national population studies give us confidence.

But also when we conduct well-done intervention studies, and increase people's omega-3 intake, we see tremendous treatment effects. One of the most impressive examples is a study published in Taiwan in 2008, in which women who had depression during pregnancy were given large amounts of omega-3 fatty acids. There was a strikingly large reduction in the severity of depression.

The core insight is that omega-3 fatty acids should be treated as an essential nutrient. If you're not getting enough omega-3, you're going to be at risk for a number of major illnesses, including heart disease. When the brain is deficient in omega-3s, you're at greater risk for whatever you're vulnerable to, such as major depression, anxiety, and perhaps unhappiness.

Fish is a complete, whole food, and it has many other beneficial nutrients. Although there is less omega-3 fatty acid in canned tuna versus fresh tuna, it is still one of the world's richest sources of omega-3s.

There is some loss of omega-3 fatty acids depending on how fish is cooked. Generally you want to avoid deep-frying it. Sardines are a great source, because they contain a huge amount of other beneficial nutrients as well. You can grind up sardines and put them in a tomato sauce and you hardly know that they're there.

You may ask, are omega-3s a wonder drug, or am I a huckster on this issue? It's important to know that I am a commissioned officer in the United States Public Health Service. I do not work for any company. I do not have any economic vested interest in selling omega-3 fatty acids. My duty is to perform scientific work that promotes the public health.

The best animal data clearly indicate that when animals are deficient in omega-3 fatty acids, it substantially depletes levels of dopamine in the

(continued)

brain. Burst releases of dopamine are critical for the experience of reward and happiness in all species. That's part of the biochemical underpinning. We haven't proven that yet in humans, but we think it goes in that direction.

The benefit is probably best described by studies in the Inuit population, where people with the highest levels of omega-3 fatty acids are the most happy.

There appears to be no upper limit to the benefits. The spectrum of emotional states affected by omega-3 fatty acids may reach from the deepest existential despair to the most sublime poetic expression of spiritual happiness. ❧

CHAPTER 6

A Journey
of the Soul

Happiness comes from the health of the soul.

AESCHYLUS, 458 BC

I have been on a spiritual journey for most of my life, and it has taken some amazing turns.

I was baptized as a Roman Catholic and raised in the Catholic tradition.

When I was an altar boy, a priest made a pass at me. In the church vestibule, as we prepared to serve mass, he started putting his hands on me. I recoiled and said, "Hey—*stop!*"

I was only twelve years old but I was almost a full six feet tall, so he backed off. I was overwhelmed with utter confusion, complete shock, and sheer disgust. In my child's mind, it was the foulest imaginable collision between God and perverted sex, like some unspeakable nightmare. I threw my altar boy outfit on the floor and bolted out of the church, never to return.

In that moment, I stopped being a religious person, in the sense that I had little further interest in organized religion and its external trappings. It shattered in my mind any illusion that priests or other clergy were anything other than highly fallible human beings.

I have great respect for people who find organized religion to be a meaningful, rewarding, and glorious part of their lives. It can be one of the ultimate powerful forces for good in this world.

For me personally, a quote from Leo Tolstoy's book *The Kingdom of God Is Within You* sums up my feeling toward the trappings of religion: "Nowhere nor in anything, except in the assertion of the Church, can we find that God or Christ founded anything like what churchmen understand by the Church." I've never read anything in any religious text that says we need a go-between between us and God, a layer of people to interpret the message or take our money.

So I don't get up every Sunday morning and go to church.

But in an unexpected way, I eventually became a deeply spiritual person, and today, spirituality is an intensely inspiring part of my daily life. It is a magnificent pathway for my happiness and for living well emotionally. Religion and spirituality are closely intertwined but they're not exactly the same thing.

One expert described religion as an *organized system* of beliefs, rituals, and symbols designed to facilitate closeness to the sacred, transcendent, or ultimate truth/reality; and spirituality as a *personal quest* for understanding the ultimate questions about life, meaning, and relationships with the sacred or transcendent, which may or may not be based in religious rituals. I don't observe the rituals, but I've been on a lifelong personal quest for understanding, so I consider myself a spiritual person.

Starting when I was in the U.S. Naval Academy and up until today, I have immersed myself in spiritual reading and thinking. After the Academy, I started reading the Bible every day. I took Bible lessons. I read the New Testament and the Psalms every day for years. I studied the Koran. I studied Buddhism, and was struck by how it parallels many of the core messages of Jesus Christ. I remembered the words of Albert Einstein when he once predicted the rise of Buddhism in the United States. "The religion of the future will be a cosmic religion," he wrote. "It should transcend personal God and avoid dogma and theology. Covering both the natural and the spiritual, it should be based on a religious sense arising from the experience of all things natural and spiritual as a meaningful unity. Buddhism answers this description."

Recently, I've been reading the key books of Jewish mystical tradition, or Kabbalah because I find some of the core readings and messages are absolutely inspiring.

In my life, I've decided to search for wisdom in all the world's spiritual traditions.

My philosophy is in line with that of the Dalai Lama when he wrote, "A variety of religions is actually necessary and useful, and therefore the only sensible thing is that all different religions work together and live harmoniously, helping one another." As Mahatma Gandhi put it, "I am a Hindu. I am a Muslim. I am a Jew. I am a Christian. I am, after all, a human being, and I am connected to all my fellow human beings!"

I pray three times a day.

I pray to thank God for all the tools and abilities that I have, and to ask God to help me make the best use of them. It took me until age fifty to do this as a really rigorous discipline. It lifts me up and makes me happy, and helps forestall or reduce any negative feelings that may creep into my day. It feels like I'm kicking off my "spiritual endorphins." I like to believe the words of Jesus Christ when he said in the Gospel of Mark 11:24:

Therefore I tell you, whatever you ask for in prayer, believe that you have received it, and it will be yours.

I believe that in our public schools there should be a period of silence every day for our children to reflect on something bigger than themselves.

We can call it a Daily Moment of Reflection.

I don't care what that something is—for different children it could be God, or spirituality, or religion, or the wonders of nature and science. Many kids have no opportunity to reflect on anything but the here and now, and we should help them take time every day to think about something larger than themselves. We should encourage them to look, as II Corinthians 4:16–18 reads, "not to things that are seen but things that are unseen."

> *The truth is that you are always united with the Lord.*
> *But you must know this.*
> *Nothing further is there to know.*
>
> HINDU SCRIPTURE, THE *UPANISHADS*

Not only can being connected to God or a greater power or to universal truths, I believe, give you happiness, joy, and peace, but there is a growing body of evidence that being religious or spiritual confers real health advantages, including mental health benefits.

That's not to say that atheists and agnostics don't have every right and ability to be happy, but being religious and/or spiritual does give many people a tremendous uplift, including myself. The research isn't perfect, and it has its critics, but many studies have reported the connections. "The evidence is unmistakable and among folks so inclined, being religious or spiritual is associated with all sorts of good outcomes," said the psychology professor Chris Peterson of the University of Michigan. He added an important qualifier: "You have to internalize it. We're not talking about Sunday Christians here; we're talking about people who live it."

Here are some of the most interesting research findings:

- A 1999 review by researchers at the National Institute for Healthcare Research examined the association of religion with depressive symptoms or depressive disorder. They found that "people with high levels of general religious involvement, organizational religious involvement, religious salience, and intrinsic religious motivation are at reduced risk for depressive symptoms and depressive disorders." They concluded that "some forms of religious involvement might exert a protective effect against the incidence and persistence of depressive symptoms or disorders."

- In his 2001 book, *The Psychology of Happiness*, the English social psychologist Michael Argyle wrote that "Religion produces positive effects on subjective well-being, especially on existential well-being but also in general happiness, mental and physical health." He credited the strong social support provided by church groups, and the ability of religion to provide meaning and purpose in life.

- Dr. David Larson of the International Center for the Integration of Health and Spirituality and his colleagues found a strong pattern in research that identified spirituality as a positive factor in helping to prevent sickness, cope with it, and treat it.

- Spiritual or religious people have been reported to suffer less depression, suicide, alcohol and drug abuse than others; as well as less hypertension, lower cholesterol levels, improved immune function, and greater longevity.

How can religion and spirituality help make us healthier and happier?

There are many possible explanations. They may foster self-confidence and the feeling that one can influence one's own destiny. Spiritual reflection, meditation, and prayer may build peace of mind, hope, and optimism, and help people cope with depression, anxiety, and the stresses of life. Religion promotes healthful behavior like sexual discretion and limiting drug, alcohol, and tobacco use.

> *When we know what the ends of things are,*
> *when we understand what the final good and final evil are,*
> *we have discovered the pathway for our life and the formation of all*
> *our due actions;*
> *we have discovered, therefore, something to which to refer each*
> *case,*
> *and hence a rational way of living well, which is what everyone*
> *seeks, can be discovered and achieved.*
>
> ANTIOCHUS OF ASCALON, SECOND CENTURY BC

I have been inspired by my personal religious study and spiritual reading for many years.

In the U.S. Navy, when I was on extended submarine deployments overseas, I'd take to bed with me the holy books of the various world religions. Sleeping quarters aboard submarines, even for officers like I was, are incredibly cramped. You squeeze into a coffinlike space, enveloped in the roaring electronic hum of the vessel, and lie down a few feet from a nuclear warhead ready to fire that's capable of destroying an entire city.

I'd put the headphones on and lose myself in the New Testament, the Hebrew Scripture, the Koran, and the great holy books of as many religions as I could find, as our ship sliced through the black waters of the Atlantic and Indian oceans.

There is a concept in Zen Buddhism called a moment of transformation, or *satori*, a flash of insight that offers a glimpse of new worlds of consciousness. When reading the great religious works, these moments seemed to come fast and furious to me.

As I journeyed a thousand feet under the surface of the ocean, and up until today, the words of Christ, and Mohammad, and Buddha, and the other great religious and wisdom figures have spoken to me across the ages.

Sometimes it feels like they are engaged in a magnificent discussion, supporting and building on each other's ideas. On occasion they seem to quote each other almost word for word!

One of the eternal truths they all seem to agree on is that the greatest pathway to your happiness and salvation is not to seek joy for yourself, but for your fellow human beings—through compassion, love, mercy, and righteousness.

There are many names for this path. Jewish mystical tradition teaches of *Chesed*, or loving kindness, as one of the Sefirot, or ten divine "rays of light." One of the Hebrew texts reads, "Every single night when a person climbs into bed, his soul leaves him, to be judged before the King's Court of Justice. If deserving to endure, she is restored to this world."

Buddhist tradition also speaks of loving kindness, or *metta*, as one of the four *brahmaviharas*, or "immeasurable states" of an enlightened person, along with compassion (*karuna*), equanimity (*upeksha*), and sympathetic joy (*mudita*), or the ability to celebrate the joy of others, and be happy when others feel happy. Very similar strains can be found in the works of Christianity, Hinduism, Islam, and other faith traditions.

A life of peace and love and joy, both here and in the worlds to come, they tell us, is possible when we seek it for others.

THE GREAT PARADOX OF THE SOUL

The Key to Achieving Happiness for Yourself
Is to Achieve Happiness for Others.

The Words of Jesus Christ

Do unto others as you would have them do unto you.

How happy are the poor in spirit, theirs is the kingdom of heaven . . .
Happy those who hunger and thirst for what is right; they shall be satisfied . . .
Happy are those who are persecuted in the cause of right: theirs is the kingdom of heaven.

The Words of Buddha

Hard it is to understand: By giving away our food, we get more strength,
by bestowing clothing on others, we gain more beauty;
by donating abodes of purity and truth, we acquire great treasures.
There is a proper time and a proper mode in charity just as the vigorous warrior goes to battle, so is the man who is able to give.
He is like an able warrior, a champion strong and wise in action.
Loving and compassionate he gives with reverence and banishes all hatred, envy and anger.
The charitable man has found the path of salvation.

He is like the man who plants a sapling, securing thereby the
shade, the flowers, and the fruit in future years.

We reach the immortal path only by continuous acts of
kindliness
and we perfect our souls by compassion and charity.

Just as a mother would protect her only child at the risk of her
own life, even so, cultivate a boundless heart towards all beings.
Let your thoughts of boundless love pervade the whole world.

The Tibetan Book of Living and Dying

Whatever joy there is in this world,
All comes from desiring others to be happy,
And whatever suffering there is in this world,
All comes from desiring myself to be happy.

The Words of the Koran

Be they Muslims, Jews, Christians, or Sabians,
Those who believe in God and the last Day
And who do good
Have their reward with their Lord.
They have nothing to fear,
And they will not sorrow.

Anyone, male or female,
who does what is good and is faithful
will enter the Garden
and will not be oppressed at all.

Absolutely, God's allies will have nothing to fear, nor will they grieve.
They are those who believe and lead a righteous life.
For them happiness in this life, and in the Hereafter.
Such is God's inviolable law.
This is the true triumph.

You have no idea how much joy and happiness are waiting for you as a reward for your (righteous) works.

Confucius

Now the man of perfect virtue, wishing to be established himself,
seeks also to establish others; wishing to be enlarged himself,
he seeks also to enlarge others.

The Rev. Martin Luther King, Jr.

Those who are not looking for happiness are the most likely to find it,
because those who are searching forget that the surest way to be happy
is to seek happiness for others.

The Hebrew Book of Zohar, or Radiance

The blessed holy one revealed to Abraham the mystery of faith,
and when he knew the mystery of faith he knew
that he was the root and sustenance of the world,
for the sake of whom the world was created and endures,
as is written: I declare, the world is built on love.

Science, too, has stepped in to echo and support the words of the religious thinkers.

In a recent analysis of published studies on altruism and its relation to mental and physical health, published in the *International Journal of Behavioral Medicine*, a team of researchers found that "a strong correlation exists between the well-being, happiness, health, and longevity of people who are emotionally and behaviorally compassionate, so long as they are not overwhelmed by helping tasks."

There is one more great truth that I have learned from the holy books and wisdom books and from my life experience, a truth that may be the greatest secret to discovering the happiness inside yourself.

It is based on an extraordinary insight—the revelation that happiness is available right here and right now, at any time in your life, if you know how to grasp it.

And it turns out the secret is an amazingly simple one.

LIVING WELL EMOTIONALLY EXPERT
Dr. Harold G. Koenig

Dr. Harold G. Koenig is one of the world's leading experts on the connections between religion, physical health, and emotional health.

He is founding codirector of the Center for Spirituality, Theology, and Health at Duke University Medical Center. He has published extensively in the fields of mental health, geriatrics, and religion, with over three hundred scientific peer-reviewed articles and book chapters and nearly forty books in print or in preparation.

Dr. Koenig is board certified in general psychiatry, geriatric psychiatry, and geriatric medicine, and is on the faculty at Duke as Professor of Psychiatry and Behavioral Sciences, and Associate Professor of

(continued)

Medicine. He is also a registered nurse (RN). He is coeditor of Duke Medicine's Faith, Spirituality and Health, *and the former editor of the* International Journal of Psychiatry in Medicine *and of* Science and Theology News. *His latest books include* The Healing Power of Faith; The Handbook of Religion and Health; Kindness and Joy; *and* Spirituality and Medicine.

Dr. Koenig has given testimony before the U.S. Senate and the U.S. House of Representatives on the effects of religious involvement on public health. He has been nominated twice for the Templeton Prize for Progress in Religion.

There have been hundreds of studies done on the connections between religion and well-being or happiness. Approximately 80 percent find that the religious person has statistically significantly more happiness, defined as positive emotions, than the less religious person.

I would be in sad shape if I didn't have my religious beliefs to depend on.

I'd be in sad shape in many ways!

I have chronic pain syndrome. I've had it since my twenties. I have psoriatic arthritis, an inflammatory arthritis that inflames the tendon insertions into the muscles and joints. Any repetitive motion creates inflammation and pain. When I was going through my medical training, I could not write or take notes, I couldn't even hold a pencil. I had to request to use a stamp to sign my name since I couldn't hold a pen. Later, I had to use voice-activated software on the computer.

Today, when I'm traveling I still have to use a wheelchair to get through airports.

Nine months ago I was diagnosed with prostate cancer.

As a physician, that was a challenge. I had always read about prostate cancer and studied it and given diagnoses of prostate cancer to other people.

But to get my own pathology report back and see the words "adenocarcinoma of the prostate" was a big shock.

For me, having religious faith has been instrumental in transforming that pain and disability into something that's meaningful. It helps give me a centerpiece of life, a sense of meaning and a sense of hope that no matter what happens, things are going to be okay because I know that God loves me and will bring about the best no matter what the circumstances.

If it's his will for my life to end, and I know he knows the best, I have the faith that things will be okay.

I was an only child and my mom died a couple of years ago. I was very close to her. For many years I thought I would completely fold, I would die, if my mom passed away. But my religious faith created a totally smooth transition. I didn't have any depression or prolonged sadness, I didn't really even have much grief. It was extraordinary. I knew that she was in good hands.

Religion is a very powerful coping behavior. It helps people to cope with adversity, particularly situational adversity like poor physical health or loss. As a whole, and everything else being equal, religious people tend to experience less depression during difficult times than those who don't have religion as a coping resource.

Religious people who get depressed recover faster than nonreligious people who are depressed. I think it's because it's such a tremendous coping behavior. It gives people hope and meaning and purpose.

Why are religious people happier?

Many religions have a positive worldview, a positive view of understanding the world.

It is a beautiful worldview, that God has a purpose in the world and that you're part of it, that God created you in his image. You are higher in God's eyes than any of the angels, and each person is unique and special in

(continued)

God's eyes. That is an amazing worldview, to love God with your whole heart and to love your neighbor as yourself. Those are beautiful attitudes to have.

Many who believe in religion believe that when you die, you are going to go to a better place that's going to be wonderful. There will be no suffering, no pain, and no disability anymore. You will see your loved ones again, and you will be with your creator in Paradise for eternity.

These beliefs are incredible! They enhance joy and well-being and our relationships with others, help us make better decisions and reduce the stress in our lives.

It's very easy to confuse religion with just "going to church." I use a broader definition of religion that includes the many dimensions of religious involvement. Only one of those aspects is religious attendance. There is also religious experience, private religious activity, religious motivation, religious knowledge, religious belief, and religious history.

In my definition, a religious or spiritual person is one who feels strongly connected to the transcendent: a connection to God, or Jehovah, or Yahweh, or Allah, or Buddha, or to ultimate truths. Their lives are determined or their decisions are informed by their religious beliefs. It's a central part of their life.

The idea that we can go outside, look at the sky, look at the sunrise, and think, "God created us, and I know I can talk to God. And he listens!"—what an incredible worldview.

That produces a feeling even beyond happiness.

It produces joy. ∽

CHAPTER 7

Living Well Emotionally Well-Being Program

Just being alive, having a wonderful family, good friends, watching the sunrise morning after morning. That's what makes me feel good.

I think people take their lives for granted, some just haven't hit that part of their lives where they stop and say, I am such a lucky person to have the life that I have.

SGT. MICHAEL A. DIRAIMONDO
IN A LETTER HOME FROM IRAQ, 2003

Every day before I go to sleep, I ask myself a ten-word question:

What did you do today that's worth talking about tomorrow?

It means, what did you do today, and what happened to you today that was good, that was positive, that was memorable, or that made you feel happy or grateful, or made someone else feel happy?

What did you achieve today?

How did you grow?

What did you learn?

How did you help others?

What did you enjoy?

What are you grateful for?

What did you do today that's worth talking about tomorrow?

Those ten words are among the guiding principles of my life.

And what that makes me do is reflect each day on anybody that I may have wronged, been curt to, rudely looked up and down, or spoke to the wrong way, making sure that the next day I don't do the same thing. If I owe somebody an apology, I try to get it done that morning. And those ten words enable me to savor the good things that happen in my life every single day.

You and I deserve a life of love and joy, a life in which we grow, prosper, and thrive emotionally, spiritually, and physically, in which happiness is a constant companion, not an impossible dream.

There is a doorway to happiness that is available to us any day, anywhere, anytime.

It turns out that some of the greatest minds in history and the greatest researchers working today agree that one of the keys to enjoying happiness can be summed up in one simple but incredibly powerful word: gratitude.

One day in December 1945, a fifteen-year-old Egyptian boy named Abu al-Majd was digging by hand for nitrate-rich fertilizer at the base of a spectacular cliff in a dusty patch of earth three hundred miles south of Cairo, near a bend in the Nile River. He picked through the soil and uncovered a large mysterious red earthenware jar. Something was inside it.

He smashed the jar open.

A small pile of thirteen books appeared, comprising hundreds of papyrus pages, each book bound in golden brown leather.

The boy did not know it, but experts later realized he had discovered some of the oldest books ever uncovered. They dated from AD 348. Believe it or not, there were sales receipts for the papyrus that enabled the date to be pinpointed. The books were written in Coptic, an ancient language of Egyptian Christians.

One of the books, experts later deciphered, bore the startling title

The Gospel of Thomas, a book that had long been rumored by scholars to exist, but had never been found before. And the book began with the tantalizing phrase "These are the secret words that the living Jesus spoke."

Inside were 114 sayings credited to the historical figure of Jesus Christ, some of which resemble passages from the four major Christian Gospels, but others that were brand-new. If they were the actual words of Christ, he sounds at times like a Zen master, as in these passages:

What you are looking forward to has come,
but you don't know it.

You examine the face of heaven and earth,
but you have not come to know the one who is in your presence,
and you do not know how to examine the present moment.

Seek and you will find.

It will not come by watching for it.
It will not be said,
"Look, here!" or "Look, there!"

Rather, the Father's kingdom is spread out upon the earth,
and people don't see it.

What if it's true? What if God's kingdom is already here, spread out all around the earth, right in front of our eyes, and all we have to do is seek it out, reach out and touch it?

Maybe what we're searching for, the love, joy, and meaning of life, is already here, and maybe the secret is, as Thomas's Christ suggests, to "know how to examine the present moment."

Maybe we already have a multitude of things to be grateful for, *and to be happy for,* if we only remembered to stop and really savor them!

"Gratitude is at the core of all the major religions," observed Robert A. Emmons, a psychologist at the University of California, and perhaps the world's leading researcher on happiness through gratitude. "Virtually every religion emphasizes gratefulness or thanksgiving. It is part of the ethical foundations of world religions which state that people are morally obligated to give thanks to their God and to each other."

He considers gratitude to be the most crucial approach to joy and contentment in life. Why? "When life is going well, it allows us to celebrate and magnify the goodness. When life is going badly, it provides a perspective by which we can view life in its entirety."

> *Life is available only in the present moment.*
> *Happiness can only be possible in the here and now.*
>
> —BUDDHA

> *Who is rich? The one who appreciates what he has.*
>
> —THE TALMUD

> *He who binds himself to a Joy,*
> *Does the winged life destroy;*
> *He who kisses the Joy as it flies,*
> *Lives in Eternity's sunrise.*
>
> —WILLIAM BLAKE

> *The greatest thing is to give thanks for everything.*
> *He who has learned this knows what it means to live.*
> *He has penetrated the whole mystery of life:*
> *giving thanks for everything.*
>
> —DR. ALBERT SCHWEITZER

Research from my laboratory shows that there are three strategies in particular that are effective at boosting happiness.

Number one is counting your blessings, expressing gratitude to others, appreciating what you have.

The second strategy is to practice acts of kindness, generosity, philanthropy, giving the gift of your time and resources.

The third strategy is training your mind to practice optimistic and hopeful thinking, to see the glass as half full.

—Professor Sonja Lyubomirsky

Pay attention to the world in which you live.

The seeds for happiness are everywhere—in the blue sky, in the clouds,
in the face of our children.

It's a joy to walk on planet Earth. It's a joy to be alive.

You may recognize that the conditions of happiness that are already there in your life are enough. Then happiness can be instantly yours.

Please take a pen and a sheet of paper.
Go to the foot of a tree or to your writing desk and make a list of all the things that can make you happy right now: the clouds in the sky, the flowers in the garden. The children playing. . . . Your beloved ones sitting in the next room. Your two eyes in good condition. The list is endless. You have enough already to be happy now.

Every moment is an opportunity to water the seeds of happiness in yourself.
Each minute, each second of life is a miracle.

—THICH NHAT HANH,
CONTEMPORARY ZEN BUDDHIST TEACHER

I'm a fifty-two-year-old bald-headed black guy who is looking for work.

In the past year I've been fired from my job as a TV talk show host for seventeen years, literally fallen on my butt a few times, and had a number of flat-out lousy days.

I have a disease with no known cause, no cure, and no way to control the pain.

I recently learned that some of the symptoms are spreading to my face—a real challenge to someone who makes his living talking to a TV camera. Eventually this stupid disease will take away my vision, my strength, my balance, my speech, and even my memory. I have to fight a battle with the disease every day.

What in the hell do I have to be grateful for?

Actually, there is a multitude of things for me to get on my knees and thank heaven for!

I have a magnificent wife and family, who inspire me and give me superstrength and inspiration. I have great friends, business partners, and colleagues.

I have literally a world full of good friends—every day, perfect strangers greet me like a long-lost friend. This happens to me all the time, on the street, in the airport, on the elevator, everywhere. Sometimes it seems like everybody is smiling at me and saying, "Hey, Montel! You look great!" It even happens to me when I'm traveling in foreign countries where they air my TV show. A few months ago I was pumping gas at a station in rural England and a fellow came over and said, "Excuse me. Are you the chap with a chat show on the telly? I just wanted to say hello!" You should have seen the smiles on both our faces.

Every day I have spiritual reading to enjoy that nourishes my soul, healthy food to savor, and exercise to do that nourishes my body and spirit. Yes, I still get depressed, but I have control over how far I fall into the pit and how long I stay there. It's my choice and my power.

Large parts of my body are still in fighting shape—my brain, my eyes, my heart, and sometimes, especially when I'm in the gym, even my limbs, muscles, and overall strength. My senses for now are fully intact—I can savor a great piece of music, a fantastic sunrise on a soft sandy beach, or a mouthwatering meal just as well as anyone. And I still have my burning ambition to succeed and make a difference in the world, and I still hold on to a feeling I first had when I was three or four years old: "There's nobody on this planet that can stop me from doing anything I want to do, period." I believe it!

Tonight when I go to sleep I'll ask myself my favorite question. But you know what? It's only noon and already four good things have happened to me today! They may seem like everyday events in life, but when I remember to stop, reflect, and savor them, they are things that make me happy right now, things I can savor in the garden of my memory.

Here's the first good thing that happened to me today: I woke up this morning and my wife and I had a minor logistical mix-up for a few seconds. What was great is that we were able to stop and talk about it calmly and laugh a bit and move forward. There were times earlier in my life when I would have melted down over it; it might have really ticked me off, and it would have sent me into a negative direction. Instead, it turned into a really nice discussion of some books we both want to read together.

The second thing: I just had a very difficult discussion with some business partners that could've been extremely unpleasant. But I decided to turn it into something positive. There's no reason you can't pause a few seconds before you say things in anger and scream and holler. Nobody needs that. It would have been unnecessary and coun-terproductive. So I took a moment to consider and put my ego in check for a minute, and we had a really productive discussion.

The third thing: I saw some tourists huddled over a map. They looked not only lost but completely bewildered by Manhattan. I offered to give them directions. We had a nice chat for a few minutes. Then we all parted with a little taste of happiness right there on Fifty-seventh Street and Broadway.

The fourth thing: I found out the waitress at the diner where I stopped for breakfast is pregnant, so I gave her a tip, plus a "baby tip." It was a little thing that made us both happy.

Stop and savor the good things—be grateful!

Or better yet, write them down. I've got my parents doing this, plus my sister and her husband. Now I want you to do it, too. Stop at the end of the day and write down what you did that's worth talking about tomorrow.

Here are the seventeen best, most powerful, and often intercon-nected ideas I have found for living a happier life, based on the wisdom I've learned from my life experience and from the greatest minds in spirituality, psychiatry, and psychology. Very special thanks to the highly respected happiness researcher Professor David G. Myers, the author of *The Pursuit of Happiness*, for his ideas and help in putting this list together.

The Living Well Emotionally Program:
17 Powerful Tips for Living a Happier Life

1. **Celebrate Three Good Things Every Day:** Keep a personal "Gratitude Journal," and at the end of every day, write down three good things that happened to you, and why.

Gratitude may be the most powerful happiness booster of all.

It is the most promising intervention yet discovered and tested by positive psychologists, and this is a technique you can start enjoying right now.

You already know the key to happiness. Your momma told you, your grandmother told you, you know it. Stop the garbage thoughts and think positive. You have to make the conscious decision. When you get up and look in the mirror, don't say, "Oh, I hate my hair. I can't believe it's so curly." Instead, say, "Dang, I've got myself some beautiful hair. I might want to cut it, but it's beautiful. Ain't nobody gonna take that from me, 'cause it's mine!"

You can also call it mindfulness, counting your blessings, grateful thinking, a sense of wonder, or a constant appreciation for the good things in your life.

The idea of keeping a "gratitude journal" may seem too simple or quaint for you at first, but you've got to try it to believe how powerful it can be. Gratitude can help you manage stress, build positive emotions, savor your positive life experiences and achievements, and boost your self-worth. It can help you put a positive reinterpretation to a negative event or traumatic ordeal. As Professor Sonja Lyubomirsky wrote, the technique will enable you "to extract the maximum possible satisfaction and enjoyment from your current circumstances."

In recent years, research by Professors Lyubomirsky, Martin Seligman, Robert Emmons, Michael McCullough, and their colleagues has linked both mental health and physical health benefits to the specific practice of keeping a gratitude journal. Emmons in particular was surprised that the physical benefits were so strong: "People keeping gratitude journals slept a half hour more per evening, woke up more refreshed and exercised 33 percent more each week compared with persons not keeping journals."

McCullough, an associate professor of psychology and religious studies at the University of Miami, noted, "There's a natural tendency to take things for granted, but if you stop and think of all the ways you are blessed, it doesn't take long for the mind to use that as the new baseline for perceiving how happy you are."

The happiness-building benefits of keeping a gratitude journal have been tested by positive psychologists and demonstrated to have long-lasting effects. You can try these variations:

- At the end of every day, write down in a journal three good things that happened to you today and why those things occurred, or three things for which you are grateful, or three things you did today that are worth talking about tomorrow. They can range from the earth-shaking, like the birth of a child, to everyday pleasures like enjoying a sunrise, a piece of music, or a lover's kiss.
- Do it once a week, say on a Sunday night, as you think about the past week, and write down "five good things."

2. **Make a Gratitude Visit:** Write a thank-you testimonial message to someone who positively affected your life, and deliver the message to him or her.

Another promising, and I think brilliant, idea developed by Professor Seligman and his colleagues, is to think of someone who made a difference in your life, compose a detailed thank-you letter, and deliver it to that person, either in person or on the phone.

The idea is to remember someone who was especially kind to you who you never had a chance to properly thank. It could be a teacher, a neighbor, a grandparent, a mentor, a member of the clergy. Think of someone who gave you a helping hand at an im-

portant time, or gave you good advice or words of encouragement, or served as an inspiration to you.

Write a testimonial of about three hundred words thanking
the person for what he did, and drop by or call him up to read it
to him. Do this once a month for a different person.

"The remarkable thing," noted Seligman when he analyzed
the results of his research on gratitude visits, "is that people who
do this just once are measurably happier and less depressed a
month later." But he added the effect wears off after three months,
so you need to repeat the tip to keep enjoying benefits.

3. **Discover Your Signature Strengths:** Take stock of your
   core strengths and commit to using them in both old and
   new ways.

A valuable step in building your personal path to happiness is to
identify the character strengths that will help you grow and thrive.
A great way to do this is to visit the positive psychology Web site
Values in Action and take the surveys to determine your "signature character strengths" (www.viasurvey.org).

The VIA Survey has 240 questions designed to reveal individual character strengths. It takes about thirty to forty minutes
to complete, and you will get an instant report on the full range
of strengths in top-down order, including your top five signature
strengths, and a description of each strength. Developed by Dr.
Chris Peterson, whom you met earlier in this book, so far it's
been taken by some 1 million people.

The VIA Brief Strengths Test is a separate, shorter measure of
character strengths for adults.

The VIA Youth Survey for young people, ages ten to seventeen, takes about forty minutes to complete.

Once you learn your own personal signature strengths, you

can think of ways to use them more often, or how to exercise them in new ways.

4. **Put Compassion into Action:** Practice personal acts of kindness.

The wisdom of the ages, and the great religions, and the best research all agree that being good to others, being altruistic, and performing routine acts of kindness in your daily life are magnificent ways of achieving meaning and happiness in your life. I believe they can ignite "upward spirals of happiness."

They can be "random acts of kindness" or highly structured, like volunteering in a food pantry.

The rewards: you'll feel better about yourself, you'll feel capable and generous, you'll win smiles and gratitude, and you'll make the world a better place.

5. **Savor the Beauty of Little Things:** Every day, feel the joy of simple pleasures.

Life is full of small, simple pleasures and fleeting moments that can give us great joy if we focus on them.

As Ben Franklin wrote, "Human felicity is produced not so much by great pieces of good fortune that seldom happen, as by little advantages that occur every day."

The sound of a child's voice, the beauty of a flower, the rich taste of a delicious lunch, the sweetness of a chocolate bar—all are tiny doorways to momentary happiness, and they can all add up, if we take time to stop and really savor them.

"Be an experiential epicure," suggested Professor David Lykken, with "a steady diet of simple pleasures." If you "sprinkle your life" with small things that you know give you a little high, "like a good meal, working in the garden, time with friends, that will leave you happier than some grand achievement that gives you a big lift for a while."

6. **Nurture Your Social Bonds:** Give priority to close relationships.

"There is one factor that is universally associated with happiness," declared Daniel Gilbert, Professor of Psychology at Harvard University and a happiness researcher, "and it's not how much you weigh or how much you earn. The extent and quality of a person's social relationships are highly correlated with happiness."

Intimate friendships with those who care deeply about you can help you weather difficult times. Confiding is good for the soul and body. Resolve to nurture your closest relationships by not taking your loved ones for granted, by displaying to them the sort of kindness you display to others, by affirming them, by playing together and sharing together.

7. **Get Moving:** Shoot for the Living Well Emotionally Physical Activity Target.

Work toward at least thirty minutes of moderate-intensity physical activity on most days of the week. An avalanche of research reveals that aerobic exercise can relieve mild depression and anxiety as it promotes health and energy. Sound minds reside in sound bodies.

Also look into other ways of nurturing your body, like relaxation therapy, meditation, deep breathing exercises, yoga, and tai chi.

8. **Nurture Your Body:** Eat well every day with the Happiness Diet.

You can feel happier and more energetic, and fight the risks of depression and many chronic diseases, if you work toward a healthy food lifestyle pattern, combined with regular physical activity. That means you:

- Base your diet on a foundation of a rich variety of many different vegetables and fruits—especially in their unprocessed states.
- Include healthy carbohydrates from whole grains, and healthy fats and protein from foods like fish, beans, and nuts.
- Minimize saturated and trans fats, sodium, processed foods, added sugars, and cholesterol in your diet.
- Be mindful of your calories-in and calories-out, to work toward a healthy body weight.
- Don't skip meals, starve yourself, or go on fad diets.

9. **Think Positive:** Cultivate an optimistic mind-set.

Don't lose sight of dangers and risks, but focus on goals, solutions, fixing problems, expecting some mistakes and learning from them—and moving on—by having confidence in yourself and staying on track. Persevere, be persistent, and never give up. You can do it! A sense of humor about yourself and about the world helps a lot, I've found.

Take control of your time: happy people feel in control of their lives. To master your use of time, set goals and break them into daily aims. Although we often overestimate how much we will accomplish in any given day (leaving us frustrated), we generally underestimate how much we can accomplish in a year, given just a little progress every day.

Project happiness: you can sometimes "act" yourself into a happier frame of mind!

Manipulated into a smiling expression, people feel better; when they scowl, the whole world seems to scowl back. So put on a happy face. Talk as if you feel positive self-esteem, are optimistic, and are outgoing. Going through the motions can trigger the emotions.

10. **Reverse the Downward Spiral of Negative Thoughts:** Make the conscious decision to ignite an upward spiral of positive emotions.

If you feel yourself starting to plunge down in the elevator of self-doubt, of overthinking, of excessive rumination and negative self-talk, stop and think about it.

Look around for little sparks of light to hold on to. Let them feed each other, light up your outlook, and lift you out of the plunge. Specific ways to do this, as Professor Barbara Fredrickson suggested:

- Find positive meaning in adversity.
- Find positive meaning in ordinary events.
- Find positive meaning in compassionately helping others.
- Find positive meaning by feeling gratitude for simple things.

11. **Realize that enduring happiness doesn't come from material success alone.**

People adapt to changing circumstances—whether an increase in wealth or the onset of a disability. Thus, wealth is like health: its utter absence breeds misery, but on the other hand, having it (or any circumstance we long for) doesn't guarantee happiness. Buying or having lots of stuff may provide moments of pleasure but will never make you truly happy.

12. **Stay in the Flow Zone:** Seek out work and leisure that engage your skills.

Often, happy people are in a zone called flow—absorbed in tasks that challenge their skills but don't overwhelm them. The most expensive forms of leisure (for example, sitting on a yacht) often provide less flow experience than gardening, socializing, or craft work.

13. **Take time to recharge yourself:** Give your body the sleep it wants.

Happy people live active, vigorous lives yet reserve time for re-newing sleep and solitude. Many people suffer from a sleep debt, which results in fatigue, diminished alertness, and gloomy moods. Go to bed in time to get a good night's sleep, every night.

14. **Nurture Your Spiritual Self:** If you're so inclined, explore religious or spiritual belief systems.

For many people, faith provides a support community, a reason to focus beyond self, and a sense of purpose and hope. Study af-ter study finds that actively religious and spiritual people are hap-pier and that they cope better with crises.

15. **Learn to Let Go:** Practice forgiveness and letting go of anger.

Many people lose friendships and end relationships because they don't know how to say two very simple little words: "I'm sorry." People just don't know how to step up to the plate and apologize, or how to forgive others. When you learn to let go of anger and learn to forgive yourself and others, you'll allow yourself to be happier.

16. **Don't Suffer in Silence:** If you're depressed, take advantage of a professional team and professional tools.

If you think you might be depressed, seek professional help immediately, and ask your doctor or therapist about promising interventions like:

- cognitive behavioral therapy
- antidepressant medications (make sure you thoroughly educate yourself on benefits and side effects)
- light therapy
- omega-3 supplementation

17. **Realize that the key to happiness lies within you:** in your own intentional activity, in what you do and how you think.

Living Well Emotionally

Resources

National Institute of Mental Health
www.nimh.nih.gov

National Mental Health Information Center
http://mentalhealth.samhsa.gov/

Positive Psychology Web sites:
www.authentichappiness.org
www.valuesinaction.org

Partnership for Prescription Assistance
www.pparx.org

Living Well with Montel Williams Web site
www.livingwellwithmontel.com/

Montel Williams MS Foundation
www.montelms.org/

Appendix 1

LIVING WELL EMOTIONALLY
FACTS AND TIPS ON MANAGING DEPRESSION
From the National Institute of Mental Health

What is depression?
Everyone occasionally feels blue or sad, but these feelings are usually fleeting and pass within a couple of days. When a person has a depressive disorder, it interferes with daily life, normal functioning, and causes pain for both the person with the disorder and those who care about him or her. Depression is a common but serious illness, and most who experience it need treatment to get better.

Many people with a depressive illness never seek treatment. But the vast majority, even those with the most severe depression, can get better with treatment. Intensive research into the illness has resulted in the development of medications, psychotherapies, and other methods to treat people with this disabling disorder.

What are the different forms of depression?
There are several forms of depressive disorders. The most common are major depressive disorder and dysthymic disorder.

Major depressive disorder, also called major depression, is characterized by a combination of symptoms that interfere with a person's ability to work, sleep, study, eat, and enjoy once-pleasurable activities. Major depression is disabling and prevents a person from functioning normally. An episode of major depression *may occur only once in a person's lifetime, but more often, it recurs throughout a person's life.*

Dysthymic disorder, also called dysthymia, is characterized by long-term (two years or longer) but less severe symptoms that may not disable a person but can prevent one from functioning normally or feeling well. People with dysthymia may also experience one or more episodes of major depression during their lifetimes.

Some forms of depressive disorder exhibit slightly different characteristics than those described above, or they may develop under unique circumstances. However, not all scientists agree on how to characterize and define these forms of depression. They include:

Psychotic depression, which occurs when a severe depressive illness is accompanied by some form of psychosis, such as a break with reality, hallucinations, and delusions.

Postpartum depression, which is diagnosed if a new mother develops a major depressive episode within one month after delivery. It is estimated that 10 to 15 percent of women experience postpartum depression after giving birth.

Seasonal affective disorder (SAD), which is characterized by the onset of a depressive illness during the winter months, when there is less natural sunlight. The depression generally lifts during spring and summer. SAD may be effectively treated with light therapy, but nearly half of those with SAD do not respond to light therapy alone. Antidepressant medication and psychotherapy can reduce SAD symptoms, either alone or in combination with light therapy.

Bipolar disorder, also called manic-depressive illness, is not as common as major depression or dysthymia. Bipolar disorder is characterized by cycling mood changes—from extreme highs (for example, mania) to extreme lows (for example, depression). Visit the National Institute of Mental Health (NIMH) Web site for more information about bipolar disorder:

www.nimh.nih.gov/

What are the symptoms of depression?

People with depressive illnesses do not all experience the same symptoms. The severity, frequency, and duration of symptoms will vary depending on the individual and his or her particular illness.

Symptoms include:

- persistent sad, anxious, or "empty" feelings
- feelings of hopelessness and/or pessimism
- feelings of guilt, worthlessness, and/or helplessness
- irritability, restlessness
- loss of interest in activities or hobbies once pleasurable, including sex
- fatigue and decreased energy
- difficulty concentrating, remembering details, and making decisions
- insomnia, early-morning wakefulness, or excessive sleeping
- overeating, or appetite loss
- thoughts of suicide, suicide attempts
- persistent aches or pains, headaches, cramps, or digestive problems that do not ease even with treatment

What illnesses often coexist with depression?

Depression often coexists with other illnesses. Such illnesses may precede the depression, cause it, and/or be a consequence of it. It is likely that the mechanics behind the intersection of depression and other illnesses differ for every person and situation. Regardless, these other co-occurring illnesses need to be diagnosed and treated.

Anxiety disorders, such as posttraumatic stress disorder (PTSD), obsessive-compulsive disorder, panic disorder, social phobia, and generalized anxiety disorder, often accompany depression. People experiencing PTSD are especially prone to having co-occurring depression. PTSD is a debilitating condition that can result after a person experiences a terrifying event or ordeal, such as a violent assault, a natural disaster, an accident, terrorism, or military combat.

People with PTSD often relive the traumatic event in flashbacks, memories, or nightmares. Other symptoms include irritability, anger outbursts, intense guilt, and avoidance of thinking or talking about the traumatic ordeal. In a National Institute of Mental Health–funded study, researchers found that more than 40 percent of people with PTSD also had depression at one-month and four-month intervals after the traumatic event.

Alcohol and other substance abuse or dependence may also co-occur with depression. In fact, research has indicated that the coexistence of mood disorders and substance abuse is pervasive among the U.S. population.

Depression also often coexists with other serious medical illnesses, such as heart disease, stroke, cancer, HIV/AIDS, diabetes, and Parkinson's disease. Studies have shown that people who have depression in addition to another serious medical illness tend to have more severe symptoms of both depression and the medical illness, more difficulty adapting to their medical condition, and more medical costs than those who do not have coexisting depression. Research has yielded increasing evidence that treating the depression can also help improve the outcome of treating the co-occurring illness.

What causes depression?

There is no single known cause of depression. Rather, it likely results from a combination of genetic, biochemical, environmental, and psychological factors.

Research indicates that depressive illnesses are disorders of the brain. Brain-imaging technologies, such as magnetic resonance imaging (MRI), have shown that the brains of people who have depression look different from those of people without depression. The parts of the brain responsible for regulating mood, thinking, sleep, appetite, and behavior appear to function abnormally. In addition, important neurotransmitters—chemicals that brain cells use to communicate—appear to be out of balance. But these images do not reveal why the depression has occurred.

Some types of depression tend to run in families, suggesting a genetic link. However, depression can occur in people without family histories of depression as well. Genetics research indicates that risk for depression results from the influence of multiple genes acting together with environmental or other factors.

In addition, trauma, loss of a loved one, a difficult relationship, or any stressful situation may trigger a depressive episode. Subsequent depressive episodes may occur with or without an obvious trigger.

How do women experience depression?

Depression is more common among women than among men. Biological, life cycle, hormonal, and psychosocial factors unique to women may be linked to women's higher depression rate. Researchers have shown that hormones directly affect brain chemistry that controls emotions and mood. For example, women are particularly vulnerable to depression after giving birth, when hormonal and physical changes, along with the new responsibility of caring for a newborn, can be overwhelming. Many new mothers experience a brief episode of the "baby blues," but some will develop postpartum depression, a much more serious condition that requires active treatment and emotional support for the new mother. Some studies suggest that women who experience postpartum depression often have had prior depressive episodes.

Some women may also be susceptible to a severe form of premenstrual syndrome (PMS), sometimes called premenstrual dysphoric disorder (PMDD), a condition resulting from the hormonal changes that typically occur around ovulation and before menstruation begins. During the transition into menopause, some women experience an increased risk for depression. Scientists are exploring how the cyclical rise and fall of estrogen and other hormones may affect the brain chemistry that is associated with depressive illness.

Finally, many women face the additional stresses of work and home responsibilities, caring for children and aging parents, abuse, poverty, and relationship strains. It remains unclear why some women faced with enormous challenges develop depression, while others with similar challenges do not.

How do men experience depression?

Men often experience depression differently from women and may have different ways of coping with the symptoms. Men are more likely to acknowledge having fatigue, irritability, loss of interest in once-pleasurable activities, and sleep disturbances, whereas women are more likely to admit to feelings of sadness, worthlessness, and/or excessive guilt.

Men are more likely than women to turn to alcohol or drugs when they are depressed, or become frustrated, discouraged, irritable, angry, and sometimes abusive. Some men throw themselves into their work to avoid talking about their depression with family or friends, or engage in reckless, risky behavior. And even though more women attempt suicide, many more men die by suicide in the United States.

How do older adults experience depression?

Depression is not a normal part of aging, and studies show that most seniors feel satisfied with their lives, despite increased physical ailments. However, when older adults do have depression, it may be overlooked because seniors may show different, less obvious symptoms, and may be less inclined to experience or acknowledge feelings of sadness or grief.

In addition, older adults may have more medical conditions, such as heart disease, stroke, or cancer, which may cause depressive symptoms, or they may be taking medications with side effects that contribute to depression. Some older adults may experience what some doctors call vascular depression, also called arteriosclerotic depression or subcortical ischemic depression. Vascular depression may result when blood vessels become less flexible and harden over time, becoming constricted. Such hardening of vessels prevents normal blood flow to the body's organs, including the brain. Those with vascular depression may have, or be at risk for, a coexisting cardiovascular illness or stroke.

Although many people assume that the highest rates of suicide are among the young, older white males age eighty-five and older actually have the highest suicide rate. Many have a depressive illness that their doctors may not detect, despite the fact that these suicide victims often visit their doctors within one month of their deaths.

The majority of older adults with depression improve when they receive treatment with an antidepressant, psychotherapy, or a combination of both. Research has shown that medication alone and combination treatment are both effective in reducing the rate of depressive recurrences in older adults. Psychotherapy alone also can be effective in prolonging periods free of depression, especially for older adults with minor depression, and it is particularly useful for those who are unable or unwilling to take antidepressant medication.

How do children and adolescents experience depression?
Scientists and doctors have begun to take seriously the risk of depression in children. Research has shown that childhood depression often persists, recurs, and continues into adulthood, especially if it goes untreated. The presence of childhood depression also tends to be a predictor of more severe illnesses in adulthood.

A child with depression may pretend to be sick, refuse to go to school, cling to a parent, or worry that a parent may die. Older children may sulk, get into trouble at school, be negative and irritable, and feel misunderstood. Because these signs may be viewed as normal mood swings typical of children as they move through developmental stages, it may be difficult to accurately diagnose a young person with depression.

Before puberty, boys and girls are equally likely to develop depressive disorders. By age fifteen, however, girls are twice as likely as boys to have experienced a major depressive episode.

Depression in adolescence comes at a time of great personal change—when boys and girls are forming an identity distinct from their parents, grappling with gender issues and emerging sexuality, and making decisions for the first time in their lives. Depression in adolescence frequently co-occurs with other disorders, such as anxiety, disruptive behavior, eating disorders, or substance abuse. It can also lead to increased risk for suicide.

An NIMH-funded clinical trial of 439 adolescents with major depression found that a combination of medication and psychotherapy was the most effective treatment option. Other NIMH-funded researchers are developing and testing ways to prevent suicide in children and adolescents, including early diagnosis and treatment, and a better understanding of suicidal thinking.

How is depression detected and treated?

Depression, even the most severe cases, is a highly treatable disorder. As with many illnesses, the earlier that treatment can begin, the more effective it is and the greater the likelihood that recurrence can be prevented.

The first step to getting appropriate treatment is to visit a doctor. Certain medications, and some medical conditions, such as viruses or a thyroid disorder, can cause the same symptoms as depression. A doctor can rule out these possibilities by conducting a physical examination, interview, and lab tests. If the doctor can eliminate a medical condition as a cause, he or she should conduct a psychological evaluation or refer the patient to a mental health professional.

The doctor or mental health professional will conduct a complete diagnostic evaluation. He or she should discuss any family history of depression, and get a complete history of symptoms—for example, when they started, how long they have lasted, their severity, and whether they have occurred before, and if so, how they were treated. He or she should also ask if the patient is using alcohol or drugs, and whether the patient is thinking about death or suicide.

Once diagnosed, a person with depression can be treated with a number of methods. The most common treatments are medication and psychotherapy.

Medication

Antidepressants work to normalize naturally occurring brain chemicals called neurotransmitters, notably serotonin and norepinephrine. Other antidepressants work on the neurotransmitter dopamine. Scientists studying depression have found that these particular chemicals are involved in regulating mood, but they are unsure of the exact ways in which they work.

The newest and most popular types of antidepressant medications are called selective serotonin reuptake inhibitors (SSRIs). SSRIs include fluoxetine (Prozac), citalopram (Celexa), sertraline (Zoloft), and several others. Serotonin and norepinephrine reuptake inhibitors (SNRIs) are similar to SSRIs and include venlafaxine (Effexor) and duloxetine (Cymbalta). SSRIs and SNRIs are more popular than the older classes of antidepressants, such as tricyclics—named for their chemical structure—and monoamine oxidase inhibitors (MAOIs) because they tend to have fewer side effects. However, medications affect everyone differently—no one-size-fits-all approach to medication exists. Therefore, for some people, tricyclics or MAOIs may be the best choice.

People taking MAOIs must adhere to significant food and medicinal restrictions to avoid potentially serious interactions. They must avoid certain foods that contain high levels of the chemical tyramine, which is found in many cheeses, wines, and pickles, and some medications, including decongestants. MAOIs interact with tyramine in such a way that may cause a sharp increase in blood pressure, which could lead to a stroke. A doctor should give a patient taking an MAOI a complete list of prohibited foods, medicines, and substances.

For all classes of antidepressants, patients must take regular doses for at least three to four weeks before they are likely to experience a full therapeutic effect. They should continue taking the medication for the time specified by their doctor, even if they are feeling better, in order to prevent a relapse of the depression. Medication should be stopped only under a doctor's supervision. Some medications need to be gradually stopped to give the body time to adjust. Although antidepressants are not habit-forming or addictive, abruptly ending an antidepressant can cause withdrawal symptoms or lead to a relapse. Some individuals, such as those with chronic or recurrent depression, may need to stay on the medication indefinitely.

In addition, if one medication does not work, patients should be open to trying another. NIMH-funded research has shown that patients who did not get well after taking a first medication increased their chances of becoming symptom-free after they switched to a different medication or added another medication to their existing one.

Sometimes stimulants, antianxiety medications, or other medications are used in conjunction with an antidepressant, especially if the patient has a coexisting mental or physical disorder. However, neither antianxiety medications nor stimulants are generally effective against depression when taken alone, and both should be taken only under a doctor's close supervision.

What are the side effects of antidepressants?
Antidepressants may cause mild and often temporary side effects in some people, but they are usually not long-term. However, any unusual reactions or side effects that interfere with normal functioning should be reported to a doctor immediately.

The most common side effects associated with SSRIs and SNRIs include:

- Headache—usually temporary and will subside.
- Nausea—temporary and usually short-lived.
- Insomnia and nervousness (trouble falling asleep or waking often during the night)—may occur during the first few weeks but often subside over time or if the dose is reduced.
- Agitation (feeling jittery).
- Sexual problems—both men and women can experience sexual problems, including reduced sex drive, erectile dysfunction, delayed ejaculation, or inability to have an orgasm.
  Tricyclic antidepressants also can cause side effects, including:
  ‣ Dry mouth—it is helpful to drink plenty of water, chew gum, and clean teeth daily.
  ‣ Constipation—it is helpful to eat more bran cereals, prunes, fruits, and vegetables.

- Bladder problems—emptying the bladder may be difficult, and the urine stream may not be as strong as usual. Older men with enlarged prostate conditions may be more affected. The doctor should be notified if it is painful to urinate.
- Sexual problems—sexual functioning may change, and side effects are similar to those from SSRIs.
- Blurred vision—often passes soon and usually will not require a new corrective lenses prescription.
- Drowsiness during the day—usually passes soon, but driving or operating heavy machinery should be avoided while drowsiness occurs. The more sedating antidepressants are generally taken at bedtime to help sleep and minimize daytime drowsiness.

FDA Warning on Antidepressants

Despite the relative safety and popularity of SSRIs and other antidepressants, some studies have suggested that they may have unintentional effects on some people, especially adolescents and young adults. In 2004, the Food and Drug Administration (FDA) conducted a thorough review of published and unpublished controlled clinical trials of antidepressants that involved nearly forty-four hundred children and adolescents. The review revealed that 4 percent of those taking antidepressants thought about or attempted suicide (although no suicides occurred), compared to 2 percent of those receiving placebos.

This information prompted the FDA, in 2005, to adopt a "black box" warning label on all antidepressant medications to alert the public about the potential increased risk of suicidal thinking or attempts in children and adolescents taking antidepressants. In 2007, the FDA proposed that makers of all antidepressant medications extend the warning to include young adults up through age twenty-four. A "black box" warning is the most serious type of warning on prescription drug labeling.

The warning emphasizes that patients of all ages taking antidepressants should be closely monitored, especially during the initial weeks of treatment. Possible side effects to look for are worsening depression, suicidal thinking or behavior, or any unusual changes in behavior, such as sleeplessness, agitation, or withdrawal from normal social situations. The warning adds that families and caregivers should also be told of the need for close monitoring and report any changes to the physician. The latest information from the FDA can be found on their Web site at www.fda.gov.

Results of a comprehensive review of pediatric trials conducted between 1988 and 2006 suggested that the benefits of antidepressant medications likely outweigh their risks to children and adolescents with major depression and anxiety disorders. The study was funded in part by the National Institute of Mental Health.

Also, the FDA issued a warning that combining an SSRI or SNRI antidepressant with one of the commonly used "triptan" medications for migraine headache could cause a life-threatening "serotonin syndrome," marked by agitation, hallucinations, elevated body temperature, and rapid changes in blood pressure. Although most dramatic in the case of the MAOIs, newer antidepressants may also be associated with potentially dangerous interactions with other medications.

What about Saint-John's-wort?
The extract from Saint-John's-wort (*Hypericum perforatum*), a bushy, wild-growing plant with yellow flowers, has been used for centuries in many folk and herbal remedies. Today in Europe, it is used extensively to treat mild to moderate depression. In the United States, it is one of the top-selling botanical products.

To address increasing American interest in Saint-John's-wort, the

National Institutes of Health conducted a clinical trial to determine the effectiveness of the herb in treating adults who have major depression. Involving 340 patients diagnosed with major depression, the eight-week trial randomly assigned one-third of them to a uniform dose of Saint-John's-wort, one-third to a commonly prescribed SSRI, and one-third to a placebo. The trial found that Saint-John's-wort was no more effective than the placebo in treating major depression. Another study is looking at the effectiveness of Saint-John's-wort for treating mild or minor depression.

Other research has shown that Saint-John's-wort can interact unfavorably with other medications, including those used to control HIV infection. On February 10, 2000, the FDA issued a Public Health Advisory letter stating that the herb appears to interfere with certain medications used to treat heart disease, depression, seizures, certain cancers, and organ transplant rejection. The herb also may interfere with the effectiveness of oral contraceptives. Because of these potential interactions, patients should always consult with their doctors before taking any herbal supplement.

Psychotherapy
Several types of psychotherapy—or "talk therapy"—can help people with depression.

Some regimens are short-term (ten to twenty weeks) and other regimens are longer-term, depending on the needs of the individual. Two main types of psychotherapies—cognitive behavioral therapy (CBT) and interpersonal therapy (IPT)—have been shown to be effective in treating depression. By teaching new ways of thinking and behaving, CBT helps people change negative styles of thinking and behaving that may contribute to their depression. IPT helps people understand and work through troubled personal relationships that may cause their depression or make it worse.

For mild to moderate depression, psychotherapy may be the best treatment option. However, for major depression or for certain people, psychotherapy may not be enough. Studies have indicated that for adolescents, a combination of medication and psychotherapy may be the most effective approach to treating major depression and reducing the likelihood for recurrence. Similarly, a study examining depression treatment among older adults found that patients who responded to initial treatment of medication and IPT were less likely to have recurring depression if they continued their combination treatment for at least two years.

Electroconvulsive Therapy
For cases in which medication and/or psychotherapy does not help alleviate a person's treatment-resistant depression, electroconvulsive therapy (ECT) may be useful. ECT, formerly known as "shock therapy," once had a bad reputation. But in recent years, it has greatly improved and can provide relief for people with severe depression who have not been able to feel better with other treatments.

Before ECT is administered, a patient takes a muscle relaxant and is put under brief anesthesia. He or she does not consciously feel the electrical impulse administered in ECT. A patient typically will undergo ECT several times a week, and often will need to take an antidepressant or mood-stabilizing medication to supplement the ECT treatments and prevent relapse. Although some patients will need only a few courses of ECT, others may need maintenance ECT, usually once a week at first, then gradually decreasing to monthly treatments for up to one year.

ECT may cause some short-term side effects, including confusion, disorientation, and memory loss. But these side effects typically clear soon after treatment. Research has indicated that after one year of ECT treatments, patients showed no adverse cognitive effects.

What efforts are under way to improve treatment?

Researchers are looking for ways to better understand, diagnose, and treat depression among all groups of people. New potential treatments are being tested that give hope to those who live with depression that is particularly difficult to treat, and researchers are studying the risk factors for depression and how it affects the brain.

How can I help a friend or relative who is depressed?

If you know someone who is depressed, it affects you, too. The first and most important thing you can do to help a friend or relative who has depression is to help him or her get an appropriate diagnosis and treatment. You may need to make an appointment on behalf of your friend or relative and go with him or her to see the doctor. Encourage him or her to stay in treatment, or to seek different treatment if no improvement occurs after six to eight weeks.

To Help a Friend or Relative

- Offer emotional support, understanding, patience, and encouragement.
- Engage your friend or relative in conversation, and listen carefully.
- Never disparage feelings your friend or relative expresses, but point out realities and offer hope.
- Never ignore comments about suicide, and report them to your friend's or relative's therapist or doctor.
- Invite your friend or relative out for walks, outings, and other activities. Keep trying if he or she declines, but don't push him or her to take on too much too soon. Although diversions and company are needed, too many demands may increase feelings of failure.
- Remind your friend or relative that with time and treatment, the depression will lift.

How can I help myself if I am depressed?

If you have depression, you may feel exhausted, helpless, and hopeless. It may be extremely difficult to take any action to help yourself. But it is important to realize that these feelings are part of the depression and do not accurately reflect actual circumstances. As you begin to recognize your depression and begin treatment, negative thinking will fade.

To Help Yourself

- Engage in mild activity or exercise. Go to a movie, a ball game, or another event or activity that you once enjoyed. Participate in religious, social, or other activities.
- Set realistic goals for yourself.
- Break up large tasks into small ones, set some priorities, and do what you can as you can.
- Try to spend time with other people and confide in a trusted friend or relative. Try not to isolate yourself, and let others help you.
- Expect your mood to improve gradually, not immediately. Do not expect to suddenly "snap out of" your depression. Often during treatment for depression, sleep and appetite will begin to improve before your depressed mood lifts.
- Postpone important decisions, such as getting married or divorced or changing jobs, until you feel better. Discuss decisions with others who know you well and have a more objective view of your situation.
- Remember that positive thinking will replace negative thoughts as your depression responds to treatment.

Where can I go for help?

If you are unsure where to go for help, ask your family doctor. Others who can help are listed below.

- Mental health specialists, such as psychiatrists, psychologists, social workers, or mental health counselors
- Health maintenance organizations
- Community mental health centers
- Hospital psychiatry departments and outpatient clinics
- Mental health programs at universities or medical schools
- State hospital outpatient clinics
- Family services, social agencies, or clergy
- Peer support groups
- Private clinics and facilities
- Employee assistance programs
- Local medical and/or psychiatric societies
- You can also check the phone book under "mental health," "health," "social services," "hotlines," or "physicians" for phone numbers and addresses. An emergency room doctor also can provide temporary help and can tell you where and how to get further help.

What if I or someone I know is in crisis?

- If you are thinking about harming yourself, or know someone who is, tell someone who can help immediately.
- Call your doctor.
- Call 911 or go to a hospital emergency room to get immediate help or ask a friend or family member to help you do these things.
- Call the toll-free, 24-hour hotline of the National Suicide Prevention Lifeline at 1-800-273-TALK (8255); TTY: 1-800-799-4TTY (4889) to talk to a trained counselor.
- Make sure you or the suicidal person is not left alone.
- Please check the NIMH Web site for the most up-to-date information on this topic.

Psychotherapies: What is psychotherapy?

Psychotherapy, or "talk therapy," is a way to treat people with a mental disorder by helping them understand their illness. It teaches people strategies and gives them tools to deal with stress and unhealthy thoughts and behaviors. Psychotherapy helps patients manage their symptoms better and function at their best in everyday life.

Sometimes psychotherapy alone may be the best treatment for a person, depending on the illness and its severity. Other times, psychotherapy is combined with medications. Therapists work with an individual or families to devise an appropriate treatment plan.

What are the different types of psychotherapy?

Many kinds of psychotherapy exist. There is no "one-size-fits-all" approach. In addition, some therapies have been scientifically tested more than others. Some people may have a treatment plan that includes only one type of psychotherapy. Others receive treatment that includes elements of several different types. The kind of psychotherapy a person receives depends on his or her needs.

The following explains several of the most commonly used psychotherapies. However, it does not cover every detail about psychotherapy. Patients should talk to their doctor or a psychotherapist about planning a treatment that meets their needs.

Cognitive Behavioral Therapy

Cognitive behavioral therapy (CBT) is a blend of two therapies: cognitive therapy (CT) and behavioral therapy. CT was developed by the psychotherapist Aaron Beck, M.D., in the 1960s. CT focuses on a person's thoughts and beliefs, and how they influence a person's mood and actions, and aims to change a person's thinking to be more adaptive and healthy. Behavioral therapy focuses on a person's actions and aims to change unhealthy behavior patterns.

CBT helps a person focus on his or her current problems and how to solve them. Both patient and therapist need to be actively involved in this process. The therapist helps the patient learn how to identify distorted or unhelpful thinking patterns, recognize and change inaccurate beliefs, relate to others in more positive ways, and change behaviors accordingly.

CBT can be applied and adapted to treat many specific mental disorders.

CBT for depression

- Many studies have shown that CBT is a particularly effective treatment for depression, especially minor or moderate depression. Some people with depression may be successfully treated with CBT only. Others may need both CBT and medication. CBT helps people with depression restructure negative thought patterns. Doing so helps people interpret their environment and interactions with others in a positive and realistic way. It may also help a person recognize things that may be contributing to the depression and help him or her change behaviors that may be making the depression worse.

CBT for anxiety disorders

- CBT for anxiety disorders aims to help a person develop a more adaptive response to a fear. A CBT therapist may use "exposure" therapy to treat certain anxiety disorders, such as a specific phobia, posttraumatic stress disorder, or obsessive-compulsive disorder. Exposure therapy has been found to be effective in treating anxiety-related disorders. It works by helping a person confront a specific fear or memory while in a safe and supportive environment. The main goals of exposure therapy are to help the patient learn that anxiety can lessen over time and give him or her the tools to cope with fear or traumatic memories.

- A recent study sponsored by the Centers for Disease Control and Prevention concluded that CBT is effective in treating trauma-related disorders in children and teens.

CBT for bipolar disorder
- People with bipolar disorder usually need to take medication, such as a mood stabilizer. But CBT is often used as an added treatment. The medication can help stabilize a person's mood so that he or she is receptive to psychotherapy and can get the most out of it. CBT can help a person cope with bipolar symptoms and learn to recognize when a mood shift is about to occur. CBT also helps a person with bipolar disorder stick with a treatment plan to reduce the chances of relapse (for example, when symptoms return).

CBT for eating disorders
- Eating disorders can be very difficult to treat. However, some small studies have found that CBT can help reduce the risk of relapse in adults with anorexia who have restored their weight. CBT may also reduce some symptoms of bulimia, and it may also help some people reduce binge-eating behavior.

CBT for schizophrenia
- Treating schizophrenia with CBT is challenging. The disorder usually requires medication first. But research has shown that CBT, as an add-on to medication, can help a patient cope with schizophrenia. CBT helps patients learn more adaptive and realistic interpretations of events. Patients are also taught various coping techniques for dealing with "voices" or other hallucinations. They learn how to identify what triggers episodes of the illness, which can prevent or reduce the chances of relapse.
- CBT for schizophrenia also stresses skill-oriented therapies.

Patients learn skills to cope with life's challenges. The therapist teaches social, daily functioning, and problem-solving skills. This can help patients with schizophrenia minimize the types of stress that can lead to outbursts and hospitalizations.

Dialectical Behavior Therapy

Dialectical behavior therapy (DBT), a form of CBT, was developed by Marsha Linehan, Ph.D. At first, it was developed to treat people with suicidal thoughts and actions. It is now also used to treat people with borderline personality disorder (BPD). BPD is an illness in which suicidal thinking and actions are more common.

The term "dialectical" refers to a philosophic exercise in which two opposing views are discussed until a logical blending or balance of the two extremes—the middle way—is found. In keeping with that philosophy, the therapist assures the patient that the patient's behavior and feelings are valid and understandable. At the same time, the therapist coaches the patient to understand that it is his or her personal responsibility to change unhealthy or disruptive behavior.

DBT emphasizes the value of a strong and equal relationship between patient and therapist. The therapist consistently reminds the patient when his or her behavior is unhealthy or disruptive—when boundaries are overstepped—and then teaches the skills needed to better deal with future similar situations. DBT involves both individual and group therapy. Individual sessions are used to teach new skills, while group sessions provide the opportunity to practice these skills.

Research suggests that DBT is an effective treatment for people with BPD. A recent NIMH-funded study found that DBT reduced suicide attempts by half compared to other types of treatment for patients with BPD.

Interpersonal Therapy

Interpersonal therapy (IPT) is most often used on a one-on-one basis to treat depression or dysthymia (a more persistent but less severe form of depression). The current manual-based form of IPT used today was developed in the 1980s by Gerald Klerman, M.D., and Myrna Weissman, M.D.

IPT is based on the idea that improving communication patterns and the ways people relate to others will effectively treat depression. IPT helps identify how a person interacts with other people. When a behavior is causing problems, IPT guides the person to change the behavior. IPT explores major issues that may add to a person's depression, such as grief, or times of upheaval or transition. Sometimes IPT is used along with antidepressant medications.

IPT varies depending on the needs of the patient and the relationship between the therapist and patient. Basically, a therapist using IPT helps the patient identify troubling emotions and their triggers. The therapist helps the patient learn to express appropriate emotions in a healthy way. The patient may also examine relationships in his or her past that may have been affected by distorted mood and behavior. Doing so can help the patient learn to be more objective about current relationships.

Studies vary as to the effectiveness of IPT. It may depend on the patient, the disorder, the severity of the disorder, and other variables. In general, however, IPT is found to be effective in treating depression.

A variation of IPT called interpersonal and social rhythm therapy (IPSRT) was developed to treat bipolar disorder. IPSRT combines the basic principles of IPT with behavioral psychoeducation designed to help patients adopt regular daily routines and sleep/wake cycles, stick with medication treatment, and improve relationships. Research has found that when IPSRT is combined with medication, it is an effective treatment for bipolar disorder. IPSRT is as effective as other types of psychotherapy combined with medication in helping to prevent a relapse of bipolar symptoms.

Family-Focused Therapy

Family-focused therapy (FFT) was developed by David Miklowitz, Ph.D., and Michael Goldstein, Ph.D., for treating bipolar disorder. It was designed with the assumption that a patient's relationship with his or her family is vital to the success of managing the illness. FFT includes family members in therapy sessions to improve family relationships, which may support better treatment results.

Therapists trained in FFT work to identify difficulties and conflicts among family members that may be worsening the patient's illness. Therapy is meant to help members find more effective ways to resolve those difficulties. The therapist educates family members about their loved one's disorder, its symptoms and course, and how to help their relative manage it more effectively. When families learn about the disorder, they may be able to spot early signs of a relapse and create an action plan that involves all family members. During therapy, the therapist will help family members recognize when they express unhelpful criticism or hostility toward their relative with bipolar disorder. The therapist will teach family members how to communicate negative emotions in a better way. Several studies have found FFT to be effective in helping a patient become stabilized and preventing relapses.

FFT also focuses on the stress family members feel when they care for a relative with bipolar disorder. The therapy aims to prevent family members from "burning out" or disengaging from the effort. The therapist helps the family accept how bipolar disorder can limit their relative. At the same time, the therapist holds the patient responsible for his or her own well-being and actions to a level that is appropriate for the person's age.

Generally, the family and patient attend sessions together. The needs of each patient and family are different, and those needs determine the exact course of treatment. However, the main components of a structured FFT usually include:

- Family education on bipolar disorder,
- Building communication skills to better deal with stress, and
- Solving problems together as a family.
- It is important to acknowledge and address the needs of family members. Research has shown that primary caregivers of people with bipolar disorder are at increased risk for illness themselves. For example, a 2007 study based on results from the NIMH-funded Systematic Treatment Enhancement Program for Bipolar Disorder (STEP-BD) trial found that primary caregivers of participants were at high risk for developing sleep problems and chronic conditions, such as high blood pressure. However, the caregivers were less likely to see a doctor for their own health issues. In addition, a 2005 study found that 33 percent of caregivers of bipolar patients had clinically significant levels of depression.

Are psychotherapies different for children and adolescents?
Psychotherapies can be adapted to the needs of children and adolescents, depending on the mental disorder. For example, the NIMH-funded Treatment of Adolescents with Depression Study (TADS) found that CBT, when combined with antidepressant medication, was the most effective treatment over the short term for teens with major depression. CBT by itself was also an effective treatment, especially over the long term. Studies have found that individual and group-based CBT are effective treatments for child and adolescent anxiety disorders. Other studies have found that IPT is an effective treatment for child and adolescent depression.

What other types of therapies are used?
In addition to the therapies listed above, many more approaches exist. Some types have been scientifically tested more than others. Also, some

of these therapies are constantly evolving. They are often combined with more established psychotherapies. A few examples of other therapies are described here.

- **Psychodynamic therapy.** Psychodynamic psychotherapy is tied to the principles of psychoanalytic theory, which assert that a person's behavior is affected by his or her unconscious mind and past experiences. Psychodynamic therapy helps people gain greater self-awareness and understanding about their own actions. It helps patients identify and explore how their nonconscious emotions and motivations can influence their behavior. Sometimes ideas from psychodynamic therapy are interwoven with other types of therapy, like CBT or IPT, to treat various types of mental disorders. Research on psychodynamic therapy is mixed, and limited. However, a review of twenty-three high-quality clinical trials involving psychodynamic therapy found it to be as effective as other established psychotherapies.

- **Light therapy.** Light therapy is used to treat seasonal affective disorder (SAD), a form of depression that usually occurs during the autumn and winter months, when the amount of natural sunlight decreases. Scientists think SAD occurs in some people when their bodies' daily rhythms are upset by short days and long nights. Research has found that the hormone melatonin is affected by this seasonal change. Melatonin normally works to regulate the body's rhythms and responses to light and dark. During light therapy, a person sits in front of a "light box" for periods of time, usually in the morning. The box emits a full-spectrum light, and sitting in front of it appears to help reset the body's daily rhythms. Also, some research indicates that a low dose of melatonin, taken at specific times of the day, can also help treat SAD.

Other types of therapies sometimes used in conjunction with the more established therapies include:

- **Expressive or creative arts therapy.** Expressive or creative arts therapy is based on the idea that people can help heal themselves through art, music, dance, writing, or other expressive acts. One study has found that expressive writing can reduce depression symptoms among women who were victims of domestic violence. It also helps college students at risk for depression.
- **Animal-assisted therapy.** Working with animals, such as horses, dogs, or cats, may help some people cope with trauma, develop empathy, and encourage better communication. Companion animals are sometimes introduced in hospitals, psychiatric wards, nursing homes, and other places where they may bring comfort and have a mild therapeutic effect. Animal-assisted therapy has also been used as an added therapy for children with mental disorders. Research on the approach is limited, but a recent study found it to be moderately effective in easing behavioral problems and promoting emotional well-being.
- **Play therapy.** This therapy is used with children. It involves the use of toys and games to help a child identify and talk about his or her feelings, as well as establish communication with a therapist. A therapist can sometimes better understand a child's problems by watching how he or she plays. Research in play therapy is minimal.

How do I find a psychotherapist?

Your family doctor can help you find a psychotherapist. Other resources for locating services:

- If unsure where to go for help, talk to someone you trust who has experience in mental health—for example, a doctor, nurse, social worker, or religious counselor. Ask their advice on where to seek treatment. If there is a university nearby, its departments of psychiatry or psychology may offer private and/or sliding-scale fee clinic treatment options. Otherwise, check the Yellow Pages under "mental health," "health," "social services," "suicide prevention," "crisis intervention services," "hotlines," "hospitals," or "physicians" for phone numbers and addresses. In times of crisis, the emergency room doctor at a hospital may be able to provide temporary help for a mental health problem, and will be able to tell you where and how to get further help.

Listed below are the types of people and places that will make a referral to, or provide, diagnostic and treatment services.

- Family doctors
- Mental health specialists, such as psychiatrists, psychologists, social workers, or mental health counselors
- Religious leaders/counselors
- Health maintenance organizations
- Community mental health centers
- Hospital psychiatry departments and outpatient clinics
- University- or medical school–affiliated programs
- State hospital outpatient clinics
- Social service agencies
- Private clinics and facilities
- Employee assistance programs
- Local medical and/or psychiatric societies

Source: National Institute of Mental Health

Appendix 2

**TIPS FOR LIVING WELL PHYSICALLY AND
EMOTIONALLY THROUGH PHYSICAL ACTIVITY**
*From the 2008 Physical Activity Guidelines for Americans
issued by the U.S. Department of Health and Human Services*

Inactivity is putting Americans at unnecessary health risk. Inactivity among children, adolescents, and adults remains relatively high, and little progress has been made in increasing levels of physical activity among Americans.

Substantial health benefits are gained by doing physical activity, including mental health and emotional health benefits.

Guidelines

Children and Adolescents (aged 6–17)
- Children and adolescents should do one hour (60 minutes) or more of physical activity every day.
- Most of the hour or more a day should be either moderate- or vigorous-intensity aerobic physical activity.

- As part of their daily physical activity, children and adolescents should do vigorous-intensity activity on at least three days per week. They also should do muscle-strengthening and bone-strengthening activity on at least three days per week.

Adults (aged 18–64)

- Adults should do two and a half hours a week of moderate-intensity, or one hour and 15 minutes (75 minutes) a week of vigorous-intensity, aerobic physical activity, or an equivalent combination of moderate- and vigorous-intensity aerobic physical activity. Aerobic activity should be performed in episodes of at least 10 minutes, preferably spread throughout the week.
- Additional health benefits are provided by increasing to five hours (300 minutes) a week of moderate-intensity aerobic physical activity, or two and a half hours a week of vigorous-intensity physical activity, or an equivalent combination of both.
- Adults should also do muscle-strengthening activities that involve all major muscle groups performed on two or more days per week.

Older Adults (aged 65 and older)

- Older adults should follow the adult guidelines. If this is not possible due to limiting chronic conditions, older adults should be as physically active as their abilities allow. They should avoid inactivity. Older adults should do exercises that maintain or improve balance if they are at risk of falling.
- For all individuals, some activity is better than none. Physical activity is safe for almost everyone, and the health benefits of physical activity far outweigh the risks. People without diagnosed chronic conditions (such as diabetes, heart disease, or osteoarthritis) and who do not have symptoms (for example,

chest pain or pressure, dizziness, or joint pain) do not need to consult with a health care provider about physical activity.

Adults with Disabilities

- Follow the adult guidelines. If this is not possible, these persons should be as physically active as their abilities allow. They should avoid inactivity.

Children and Adolescents with Disabilities

- Work with the child's health care provider to identify the types and amounts of physical activity appropriate for them. When possible, these children should meet the guidelines for children and adolescents—or as much activity as their condition allows. Children and adolescents should avoid being inactive.

Pregnant and Postpartum Women

- Healthy women who are not already doing vigorous-intensity physical activity should get at least two and a half hours (150 minutes) of moderate-intensity aerobic activity a week. Preferably, this activity should be spread throughout the week. Women who regularly engage in vigorous-intensity aerobic activity or high amounts of activity can continue their activity provided that their condition remains unchanged and they talk to their health care provider about their activity level throughout their pregnancy.

The Scientific Evidence for the Health Benefits of Physical Activity

Adults and Older Adults

Strong Evidence:

Lower risk of:

early death

heart disease

stroke

type 2 diabetes

high blood pressure

adverse blood lipid profile

metabolic syndrome

colon and breast cancers

prevention of weight gain

weight loss when combined with diet

improved cardiorespiratory and muscular fitness

prevention of falls

reduced depression

better cognitive function (older adults)

Moderate to Strong Evidence:

better functional health (older adults)

reduced abdominal obesity

Moderate Evidence:

weight maintenance after weight loss

lower risk of hip fracture

increased bone density

improved sleep quality

lower risk of lung and endometrial cancers

Children and Adolescents

Strong Evidence:

improved cardiorespiratory endurance and muscular fitness

favorable body composition

improved bone health

improved cardiovascular and metabolic health biomarkers

Moderate Evidence:
reduced symptoms of anxiety and depression

Physical Activity Has Many Health Benefits

All Americans should be regularly physically active to improve overall health and fitness and to prevent many adverse health outcomes. The benefits of physical activity occur in generally healthy people, in people at risk of developing chronic diseases, and in people with current chronic conditions or disabilities.

Physical activity affects many health conditions, and the specific amounts and types of activity that benefit each condition vary. In developing public health guidelines, the challenge is to integrate scientific information across all health benefits and identify a critical range of physical activity that appears to have an effect across the health benefits. One consistent finding from research studies is that once the health benefits from physical activity begin to accrue, additional amounts of activity provide additional benefits.

Although some health benefits seem to begin with as little as 60 minutes a week, research shows that a total amount of 150 minutes (two hours and 30 minutes) a week of moderate-intensity aerobic activity, such as brisk walking, consistently reduces the risk of many chronic diseases and other adverse health outcomes.

Examining the Relationship Between Physical Activity and Health

In many studies covering a wide range of issues, researchers have focused on exercise as well as on the more broadly defined concept of physical activity. Exercise is a form of physical activity that is planned, structured, repetitive, and performed with the goal of improving health or fitness. So, although all exercise is physical activity, not all physical activity is exercise.

Studies have examined the role of physical activity in many groups—

men and women, children, teens, adults, older adults, people with disabilities, and women during pregnancy and the postpartum period. These studies have focused on the role that physical activity plays in many health outcomes, including:

- premature (early) death
- diseases, such as coronary heart disease, stroke, some cancers, type 2 diabetes, osteoporosis, and depression
- risk factors for disease, such as high blood pressure and high blood cholesterol
- physical fitness, such as aerobic capacity, and muscle strength and endurance
- functional capacity (the ability to engage in activities needed for daily living)
- mental health, such as depression and cognitive function
- injuries or sudden heart attacks

The Health Benefits of Physical Activity—Major Research Findings

- Regular physical activity reduces the risk of many adverse health outcomes.
- Some physical activity is better than none.
- For most health outcomes, additional benefits occur as the amount of physical activity increases through higher intensity, greater frequency, and/or longer duration.
- Most health benefits occur with at least 150 minutes a week of moderate-intensity physical activity, such as brisk walking. Additional benefits occur with more physical activity.

- Both aerobic (endurance) and muscle-strengthening (resistance) physical activity are beneficial.
- Health benefits occur for children and adolescents, young and middle-aged adults, older adults, and those in every studied racial and ethnic group.
- The health benefits of physical activity occur for people with disabilities.
- The benefits of physical activity far outweigh the possibility of adverse outcomes.

These studies have also prompted questions as to what types and how much physical activity is needed for various health benefits. To answer this question, investigators have studied three main kinds of physical activity: aerobic, muscle-strengthening, and bone-strengthening. Investigators have also studied balance and flexibility activities.

Aerobic Activity
In this kind of physical activity (also called an endurance activity or cardio activity), the body's large muscles move in a rhythmic manner for a sustained period of time. Brisk walking, running, bicycling, jumping rope, and swimming are all examples. Aerobic activity causes a person's heart to beat faster than usual.

Aerobic physical activity has three components:

- Intensity, or how hard a person works to do the activity. The intensities most often examined are moderate intensity (equivalent in effort to brisk walking) and vigorous intensity (equivalent in effort to running or jogging);
- Frequency, or how often a person does aerobic activity; and

- Duration, or how long a person does an activity in any one session.
- Although these components make up a physical activity profile, research has shown that the total amount of physical activity (minutes of moderate-intensity physical activity, for example) is more important for achieving health benefits than is any one component (frequency, intensity, or duration).

Muscle-Strengthening Activity

This kind of activity, which includes resistance training and lifting weights, causes the body's muscles to work or hold against an applied force or weight. These activities often involve relatively heavy objects, such as weights, which are lifted multiple times to train various muscle groups. Muscle-strengthening activity can also be done by using elastic bands or body weight for resistance (climbing a tree or doing push-ups, for example).

Muscle-strengthening activity also has three components:

- Intensity, or how much weight or force is used relative to how much a person is able to lift;
- Frequency, or how often a person does muscle-strengthening activity; and
- Repetitions, or how many times a person lifts a weight (analogous to duration for aerobic activity). The effects of muscle-strengthening activity are limited to the muscles doing the work. It's important to work all the major muscle groups of the body: the legs, hips, back, abdomen, chest, shoulders, and arms.

Bone-Strengthening Activity

This kind of activity (sometimes called weight-bearing or weight-loading activity) produces a force on the bones that promotes bone growth and strength. This force is commonly produced by impact with the ground. Examples of bone-strengthening activity include jumping jacks, running, brisk walking, and weight-lifting exercises. As these examples illustrate, bone-strengthening activities can also be aerobic and muscle-strengthening.

The Health Benefits of Physical Activity

Studies clearly demonstrate that participating in regular physical activity provides many health benefits. Many conditions affected by physical activity occur with increasing age, such as heart disease and cancer. Reducing the risk of these conditions may require years of participation in regular physical activity. However, other benefits, such as increased cardiorespiratory fitness, increased muscular strength, and decreased depressive symptoms and blood pressure, require only a few weeks or months of participation in physical activity.

How does physical activity increase health? It's about overload, progression, and specificity. *Overload* is the physical stress placed on the body when physical activity is greater in amount or intensity than usual. The body's structures and functions respond and adapt to these stresses. For example, aerobic physical activity places a stress on the cardiorespiratory system and muscles, requiring the lungs to move more air and the heart to pump more blood and deliver it to the working muscles. This increase in demand increases the efficiency and capacity of the lungs, heart, circulatory system, and exercising muscles. In the same way, muscle-strengthening and bone-strengthening activities overload muscles and bones, making them stronger.

Progression is closely tied to overload. Once a person reaches a certain fitness level, he or she progresses to higher levels of physical activity by continued overload and adaptation. Small, progressive changes in overload help the body adapt to the additional stresses while minimizing the risk of injury.

Specificity means that the benefits of physical activity are specific to the body systems that are doing the work. For example, aerobic physical activity largely benefits the body's cardiovascular system.

The health benefits of physical activity are seen in children and adolescents, young and middle-aged adults, older adults, women and men, people of different races and ethnicities, and people with disabilities and chronic conditions. The health benefits of physical activity are generally independent of body weight. Adults of all sizes and shapes gain health and fitness benefits by being habitually physically active. The benefits of physical activity also outweigh the risk of injury and sudden heart attacks, two concerns that prevent many people from becoming physically active.

Premature Death
Strong scientific evidence shows that physical activity reduces the risk of premature death (dying earlier than the average age of death for a specific population group) from the leading causes of death, such as heart disease and some cancers, as well as from other causes of death. This effect is remarkable in two ways:

- First, only a few lifestyle choices have as large an effect on mortality as physical activity. It has been estimated that people who are physically active for approximately seven hours a week have a 40 percent lower risk of dying early than those who are active for less than 30 minutes a week.
- Second, it is not necessary to do high amounts of activity or vigorous-intensity activity to reduce the risk of premature death. Studies show substantially lower risk when people do 150 minutes of at least moderate-intensity aerobic physical activity a week.
- Research clearly demonstrates the importance of avoiding inactivity. Even low amounts of physical activity reduce the risk of dying prematurely.

Cardiorespiratory Health

The benefits of physical activity on cardiorespiratory health are some of the most extensively documented of all the health benefits. Cardiorespiratory health involves the health of the heart, lungs, and blood vessels.

- Heart diseases and stroke are two of the leading causes of death in the United States. Risk factors that increase the likelihood of cardiovascular diseases include smoking, high blood pressure (called hypertension), type 2 diabetes, and high levels of certain blood lipids (such as low-density lipoprotein, or LDL, cholesterol). Low cardiorespiratory fitness also is a risk factor for heart disease.

- People who do moderate- or vigorous-intensity aerobic physical activity have a significantly lower risk of cardiovascular disease than do inactive people. Regularly active adults have lower rates of heart disease and stroke, and have lower blood pressure, better blood lipid profiles, and fitness. Significant reductions in the risk of cardiovascular disease occur at activity levels equivalent to 150 minutes a week of moderate-intensity physical activity. Even greater benefits are seen with 200 minutes (three hours and 20 minutes) a week. The evidence is strong that greater amounts of physical activity result in even further reductions in the risk of cardiovascular disease.

- Everyone can gain the cardiovascular health benefits of physical activity. The amount of physical activity that provides favorable cardiorespiratory health and fitness outcomes is similar for adults of various ages, including older people, as well as for adults of various races and ethnicities. Aerobic exercise also improves cardiorespiratory fitness in individuals with some disabilities, including people who have lost the use of one or both legs and those with multiple sclerosis, stroke, spinal cord injury, and cognitive disabilities.

- Moderate-intensity physical activity is safe for generally healthy women during pregnancy. It increases cardiorespiratory fitness without increasing the risk of early pregnancy loss, preterm delivery, or low birth weight. Physical activity during the post-partum period also improves cardiorespiratory fitness.

Metabolic Health

Regular physical activity strongly reduces the risk of developing type 2 diabetes as well as the metabolic syndrome. The metabolic syndrome is defined as a condition in which people have some combination of high blood pressure, a large waistline (abdominal obesity), an adverse blood lipid profile (low levels of high-density lipoprotein [HDL] cholesterol, raised triglycerides), and impaired glucose tolerance.

- People who regularly engage in at least moderate-intensity aerobic activity have a significantly lower risk of developing type 2 diabetes than do inactive people. Although some experts debate the usefulness of defining the metabolic syndrome, good evidence exists that physical activity reduces the risk of having this condition, as defined in various ways. Lower rates of these conditions are seen with 120 to 150 minutes (two hours to two hours and 30 minutes) a week of at least moderate-intensity aerobic activity. As with cardiovascular health, additional levels of physical activity seem to lower the risk even further. In addition, physical activity helps control blood glucose levels in persons who already have type 2 diabetes.
- Physical activity also improves metabolic health in youth. Studies find this effect when young people participate in at least three days of vigorous aerobic activity a week. More physical activity is associated with improved metabolic health, but research has yet to determine the exact amount of improvement.

Obesity and Energy Balance

Overweight and obesity occur when fewer calories are expended, including calories burned through physical activity, than are taken in through food and beverages. Physical activity and caloric intake both must be considered when trying to control body weight. Because of this role in energy balance, physical activity is a critical factor in determining whether a person can maintain a healthy body weight, lose excess body weight, or maintain successful weight loss. People vary a great deal in how much physical activity they need to achieve and maintain a healthy weight. Some need more physical activity than others to maintain a healthy body weight, to lose weight, or to keep weight off once it has been lost.

- Strong scientific evidence shows that physical activity helps people maintain a stable weight over time. However, the optimal amount of physical activity needed to maintain weight is unclear. People vary greatly in how much physical activity results in weight stability. Many people need more than the equivalent of 150 minutes of moderate-intensity activity a week to maintain their weight.
- Research shows that over short periods of time, such as a year, it is possible to achieve weight stability by doing the equivalent of two and a half to five hours a week of moderate-intensity walking at about a four-mile-an-hour pace. Muscle-strengthening activities may help promote weight maintenance, although not to the same degree as aerobic activity.
- People who want to lose a substantial (more than 5 percent of body weight) amount of weight and people who are trying to keep a significant amount of weight off once it has been lost need a high amount of physical activity unless they also reduce their caloric intake. Many people need to do more than five

hours of moderate-intensity activity a week to meet weight-control goals.

- Regular physical activity also helps control the percentage of body fat in children and adolescents. Exercise training studies with overweight and obese youth have shown that they can reduce their body fatness by participating in physical activity that is at least moderate intensity on three to five days a week, for 30 to 60 minutes each time.

Musculoskeletal Health

Bones, muscles, and joints support the body and help it move. Healthy bones, joints, and muscles are critical to the ability to do daily activities without physical limitations.

- Preserving bone, joint, and muscle health is essential with increasing age. Studies show that the frequent decline in bone density that happens during aging can be slowed with regular physical activity. These effects are seen in people who participate in aerobic, muscle-strengthening, and bone-strengthening physical activity programs of moderate or vigorous intensity. The range of total physical activity for these benefits varies widely. Important changes seem to begin at 90 minutes a week and continue up to 300 minutes a week.
- Hip fracture is a serious health condition that can have life-changing negative effects for many older people. Physically active people, especially women, appear to have a lower risk of hip fracture than do inactive people. Research studies on physical activity to prevent hip fracture show that participating in 120 to 300 minutes a week of physical activity that is of at least moderate intensity is associated with a reduced risk. It is unclear, however, whether activity also lowers the risk of fractures of the spine or other important areas of the skeleton.

- The bottom line is that the health benefits of physical activity far outweigh the risks of adverse events for almost everyone.
- Building strong, healthy bones is also important for children and adolescents. Along with having a healthy diet that includes adequate calcium and vitamin D, physical activity is critical for bone development in children and adolescents. Bone-strengthening physical activity done three or more days a week increases bone-mineral content and bone density in youth.
- Regular physical activity also helps people with arthritis or other rheumatic conditions affecting the joints. Participation in 130 to 150 minutes (two hours and 10 minutes to two hours and 30 minutes) a week of moderate-intensity, low-impact physical activity improves pain management, function, and quality of life. Researchers don't yet know whether participation in physical activity, particularly at low to moderate intensity, reduces the risk of osteoarthritis. Very high levels of physical activity, however, may have extra risks. People who participate in very high levels of physical activity, such as elite or professional athletes, have a higher risk of hip and knee osteoarthritis, mostly due to the risk of injury involved in competing in some sports.
- Progressive muscle-strengthening activities increase or preserve muscle mass, strength, and power. Higher amounts (through greater frequency or higher weights) improve muscle function to a greater degree. Improvements occur in younger and older adults. Resistance exercises also improve muscular strength in persons with such conditions as stroke, multiple sclerosis, cerebral palsy, spinal cord injury, and cognitive disability. Though it doesn't increase muscle mass in the same way that muscle-strengthening activities do, aerobic activity may also help slow the loss of muscle with aging.

Cancer

Physically active people have a significantly lower risk of colon cancer than do inactive people, and physically active women have a significantly lower risk of breast cancer. Research shows that a wide range of moderate-intensity physical activity—between 210 and 420 minutes a week (three hours and 30 minutes to seven hours)—is needed to significantly reduce the risk of colon and breast cancer; currently, 150 minutes a week does not appear to provide a major benefit. It also appears that greater amounts of physical activity lower the risks of these cancers even further, although exactly how much lower is not clear.

- Although not definitive, some research suggests that the risk of endometrial cancer in women and lung cancers in men and women also may be lower among those who are regularly active compared to those who are inactive.
- Finally, cancer survivors have a better quality of life and improved physical fitness if they are physically active, compared to survivors who are inactive.

Mental Health

Physically active adults have lower risk of depression and cognitive decline (declines with aging in thinking, learning, and judgment skills). Physical activity also may improve the quality of sleep. Whether physical activity reduces distress or anxiety is currently unclear.

- Mental health benefits have been found in people who do aerobic or a combination of aerobic and muscle-strengthening activities three to five days a week for 30 to 60 minutes at a time. Some research has shown that even lower levels of physical activity also may provide some benefits.
- Regular physical activity appears to reduce symptoms of anxiety and depression for children and adolescents.

Source Notes

Chapter 2: A Journey of the Mind

p. 31: "I believe that the very purpose of our life": Dalai Lama and Howard C. Cutler, *The Art of Happiness: A Handbook for Living* (London: Compass Press, 1999), p. 13.

p. 33: "The feeling that power increases": Mark Kingwell, *Better Living: In Pursuit of Happiness from Plato to Prozac* (New York: Viking, 1998), p. 4.

p. 33: "To be strong is to be happy": Burton Stevenson, *The Home Book of Proverbs, Maxims and Familiar Phrases* (New York: Macmillan, 1945), p. 1070.

p. 36: "We are in the midst of an epidemic": Will Wilkinson, "The Great Depression," *Reason*, December 2007.

p. 41: "Consider these stark statistics": National Institute of Mental Health Web site; Allan V. Horwitz and Jerome C. Wakefield, *The Loss of Sadness: How Psychiatry Transformed Normal Sorrow Into Depressive Dis-*

order (New York: Oxford University Press, 2007), pp. 4–5, 187, 215; Barbara L. Fredrickson, "The Value of Positive Emotions," *American Scientist*, July 2003; N. F. Smith, "The Elusive Affliction," *Town & Country*, May 2000; and Lynette L. Craft and Frank M. Perna, "The Benefits of Exercise for the Clinically Depressed," *Primary Care Companion to the Journal of Clinical Psychiatry* 6, 2004.

p. 42: "To call yourself happy": Stevenson, *The Home Book of Proverbs*, p. 1073.

p. 42: "Well-being and happiness never appeared": John F. Schumaker, "The Happiness Gap," *Ottawa Citizen*, October 6, 2006.

p. 42: "Ask yourself whether you are happy": Kingwell, *Better Living*, p. 4.

p. 42: "Is life satisfaction always great?": Jean Chatzky, "Want to Be Rich? Don't Be Too Happy," *Money*, June 2008.

p. 42: "unbroken happiness is a bore"; "hell on earth": Stevenson, *The Home Book of Proverbs*, p. 1073.

p. 43: "you become more analytical"; "once a moderate level of happiness"; "If you're totally satisfied": Sharon Begley, "Happiness: Enough Already," *Newsweek*, February 11, 2008.

p. 43: "Without scaling mountains": Stevenson, *The Home Book of Proverbs*, p. 1119.

p. 43: "The person who has had more experience"; "Suffering produces endurance": Jonathan Haidt, *The Happiness Hypothesis: Finding Modern Truth in Ancient Wisdom* (New York: Basic Books, 2006), p. 139.

p. 44: "These are borderline states": R. Moacanin, *Jung's Psychology and Tibetan Buddhism* (Somerville, Mass.: Wisdom Publications, 1986), p. 67.

p. 44: "There are no shortcuts. There is no 'happiness now'": Kathleen Megan, "The Pursuit of Unhappiness," *Hartford Courant,* March 2, 2008.

p. 44: "Sadness is an inherent part": Horwitz and Wakefield, *The Loss of Sadness,* p. 224.

p. 46: "The cost of not looking at context": Shankar Vedantam, "Criteria for Depression Are Too Broad, Researchers Say," *Washington Post,* April 3, 2007.

p. 53: "researchers at the University College London published some fascinating studies": A. Steptoe et al., "Positive Affect and Biological Function in Everyday Life," *Neurobiology of Aging,* December 2005; "Positive Affect and Health-related Neuroendocrine, Cardiovascular, and Inflammatory Processes," *Proceedings of the National Academy of Science,* May 2005; and "Positive Psychological Well-being and Mortality: A Quantitative Review of Prospective Observational Studies," *Psychosomatic Medicine,* September 2008.

p. 53: "Diener at the University of Illinois has found": "Contributions of the Ed Diener Laboratory to the Scientific Understanding of Well-Being," www.psych.uiuc.edu/~ediener/

p. 59: "The whole universe is change": Haidt, *The Happiness Hypothesis,* p. 23.

p. 59: "The mind is its own place": Ibid., p. 34.

p. 60:"If I am not for myself": Sonja Lyubomirsky, *The How of Happiness, A Scientific Approach to Getting the Life You Want* (New York: Penguin, 2008), p. 124.

p. 60: "It's never the events": Albert Ellis, *The Myth of Self-esteem: How Rational Emotive Behavior Therapy Can Change Your Life Forever* (Amherst, N.Y.: Prometheus Books, 2005), p. 259.

p. 60: "Happiness is life": Julia Annas, *The Morality of Happiness* (New York: Oxford University Press, 1995), p. 415.

p. 60: "O mortal men, why seek ye for happiness": Stevenson, *The Home Book of Proverbs*, p. 1070.

p. 60: "Happiness and misery depend": David G. Myers, *The Pursuit of Happiness: Who Is Happy, and Why* (New York: William Morrow, 1992), p. 105.

p. 61: "Man is the artificer": Stevenson, *The Home Book of Proverbs*, p. 1070.

p. 61: "All happiness is in the mind": Ibid., p. 1073.

p. 61: "Most people are about as happy": Edward C. Goodman, Ted Goodman, *The Forbes Book of Business Quotations: 14,266 Thoughts on the Business of Life* (New York: Black Dog & Leventhal Publishers, 1997), p. 385.

p. 61: "Happiness does not depend": John Cook, Steve Deger, Leslie Ann Gibson, *The Book of Positive Quotations* (Minneapolis: Fairview Press, 2007), p. 29.

p. 61: "To be in hell is to drift": Stevenson, *The Home Book of Proverbs*, p. 1120.

p. 61: "It is not that someone else": Thomas Merton, *New Seeds of Contemplation* (New York: New Directions, 1972), p. 110.

p. 61: "I am responsible for the achievement": Nathaniel Branden, *The Psychology of Self-Esteem* (New York: Jossey-Bass, 2001), pp. 258, 259.

Chapter 3: Seven Breakthroughs on the Road to Happiness

p. 66: The three professors, happiness formula: Sonja Lyubomirsky, Ken Sheldon, and David Schkade, "Pursuing Happiness: The Architecture of Sustainable Change," *Review of General Psychology*, 2006, p. 9.

p. 67: "Once you get basic human needs": Kyung M. Song, "The How and Why of Happiness," *Seattle Times*, February 11, 2004.

p. 67: "We're not slaves to our genes": Jenny Bailly, "Get Happy," *Allure*, February 2008.

p. 68: "Happiness is something"; "If you want to keep your happiness": Holly J. Morris, "Happiness Explained," *US News & World Report*, August 26, 2001.

p. 68: "Eight Habits of the Happiest People": Lyubomirsky, *The How of Happiness*, pp. 22, 23.

p. 72: "The idea was that if you sat back": Erica Goode, "Pragmatist Embodies His No-Nonsense Therapy," *New York Times*, January 11, 2000.

p. 73: "Depressed people are caught": Haidt, *The Happiness Hypothesis*, p. 38.

p. 74: "few academics or private psychiatrists": Cecilia Capuzzi Simon, "A Change of Mind," *Washington Post*, September 3, 2002.

p. 74: "She was just following the old road": Gail Shister, "He Shows No Signs of a Beckian Slip," *Philadelphia Inquirer*, May 11, 2008.

p. 75: "A degree in psychiatry": Andrew Solomon, *The Noonday Demon: An Atlas of Depression* (New York: Simon & Schuster, 2002), p. 106.

p. 78: "Risks and side effects of antidepressants": Dr. Richard Rosenthal points out that given the large number of adults who have taken antidepressants for severe depression, it is clear that many lives have been improved, or even saved, in spite of the risk of side effects. No medicine is free of risks, and all antidepressant treatment needs professional monitoring.

p. 79: "do not produce clinically significant improvements": Irving Kirsch et al., "Initial Severity and Antidepressant Benefits: A Meta-Analysis of Data Submitted to the Food and Drug Administration," *Philosophy, Ethics, and Humanities in Medicine*, May 27, 2008.

p. 83: "positive psychology": many of the basic ideas of the positive psychology movement were expressed in the special January 2000 issue of *American Psychologist*, edited by Martin Seligman and Mihaly Csikszentmihalyi.

p. 83: "Why can't you stop being such a grouch?": "The Sunshine Prescription," *Boston Globe*, September 22, 2002.

p. 84: "I realized that my profession"; "It wasn't enough for us"; "This is newsworthy": Claudia Wallis, "The New Science of Happiness," *Time*, January 15, 2005.

p. 84: "We've forgotten about the rest of our mission": Martin Seligman, Acacia Parks, Tracy Steen, "A Balanced Psychology and a Full Life," The Royal Society, *Philosophical Transactions: Biological Sciences*, August 18, 2004.

p. 89: "People need to learn"; "great moments in self-efficacy": Melinda Beck, "If at First You Don't Succeed," *Wall Street Journal*, April 29, 2008.

p. 90: "Every day is a new life": Dale Carnegie, *How to Stop Worrying and Start Living* (New York: Simon & Schuster, 1948), p. 7.

p. 90: "If ye have faith": Dale Carnegie, *Dale Carnegie's Scrapbook* (New York: Simon & Schuster, 1959), p. 17.

p. 91: "Our greatest glory": Ibid., p. 17.

p. 91: "Happy the Man": Ibid., p. 64.

p. 91: "For failure comes from the inside": Joseph Morris, *It Can Be Done: Poems of Inspiration* (Whitefish, Mt.: Kessinger Publishing, 2003), p. 50.

p. 91: "For every day I stand": Robert Collier, *Secret of the Ages* (St. Paul, Minn.: Wilder Publications, 2007), p. 73.

p. 91: "Finish each day": Lyubomirsky, *The How of Happiness*, p. 112.

p. 92: "Success begins with a fellow's will": Napoleon Hill, *Think and Grow Rich* (Charleston, S.C.: Forgotten Books, 1962), p. 57.

p. 92: "Courage is rightly esteemed": *Dale Carnegie's Scrapbook*, p. 18.

p. 92: "Action may not always": Ibid., p. 21.

p. 92: "The secret of being miserable": Ibid., p. 61.

p. 93: "It is not how much we have": Ibid., p. 84.

p. 93: "The secret of happiness": Ibid., p. 92.

p. 93: "To improve the golden moment": Ibid., p. 93.

p. 93: "They can conquer": Ibid., p. 8.

p. 93: "The road to failure is paved": Tiger Woods and Golf Digest, *How I Play Golf: Ryder Cup Edition* (New York: Warner Books, 2001), p. 269.

p. 93: "I've failed over and over": Beck, "If at First You Don't Succeed."

p. 98: "Rumination . . . whether rehashing things": Bailly, "Get Happy."

p. 99: "broaden and build" theory: Barbara L. Fredrickson, "The Role of Positive Emotions in Positive Psychology: The Broaden-and-Build Theory of Positive Emotions," *American Psychologist*, March 2001.

p. 99: "mutually reinforcing ascent": Barbara L. Fredrickson, "The Value of Positive Emotions," *American Scientist*, July 2003.

p. 99: "Cultivating positive emotions": "Largest Psychology Prize Ever Goes to University of Michigan Expert," *Ascribe News*, May 16, 2000.

p. 100: "Frederickson has outlined is to *find positive meaning*": Fredrickson, "The Value of Positive Emotions."

p. 101: "The happiness of a man"; "The chiefest point of happiness"; "It is neither wealth, nor splendor"; "The only happiness a brave man": Stevenson, *The Home Book of Proverbs*, p. 1070.

p. 101: "A good life is one": C. R. Snyder, Shane J. Lopez, *Handbook of Positive Psychology* (New York: Oxford University Press, 2005), p. 89.

pp. 101–02: "If you mess up"; "You're going all out"; "It almost feels like": Dave Phillips, "Flow," *Gazette* (Colorado Springs), December 14, 2007.

p. 102: "You lose your sense of time"; "being carried away"; "In many ways, the secret": Mihaly Csikszentmihalyi, "Happiness and Creativity: Going with the Flow," *Futurist*, September 19, 1997.

p. 102: "is that it involves a challenge": Mihaly Csikszentmihalyi, "The Secrets of Happiness," *Times*, September 19, 2005.

Chapter 4: A Journey of the Body

p. 111: "a growing number of studies indicate": Lesley White, Rudolph Dressendorfer, "Exercise and Multiple Sclerosis," *Sports Medicine* 34, 2004.

p. 111: "Exercise is the first step": Solomon, *The Noonday Demon*, p. 138.

p. III: "I can't overstate how important": Simon Usborne, "Train Your Brain," *Independent*, March 25, 2008.

p. 112: "A brisk five-to ten-minute walk": Bailly, "Get Happy."

p. 112: "Our results suggest": Alexander Harris et al., "Physical Activity, Exercise Coping, and Depression in a 10-year Cohort Study of Depressed Patients," *Journal of Affective Disorders,* March 2006.

p. 113: "seems generally comparable": James A. Blumenthal et al., "Exercise and Pharmacotherapy in the Treatment of Major Depressive Disorder," *Psychosomatic Medicine* 69, 2007.

p. 113: "There is certainly growing evidence": Amy Norton, "Exercise on Par with Drugs for Aiding Depression," Reuters, September 19, 2007.

p. 114: Theories for exercise effectiveness, "running has been compared": Lynette L. Craft and Frank M. Perna, "The Benefits of Exercise for the Clinically Depressed," *Primary Care Companion to the Journal of Clinical Psychiatry* 6, 2004.

p. 114: "researchers at the University of Bonn": "New Research Validates Runner's High," *Day to Day*, National Public Radio, March 31, 2008.

p. 114: "the more a person walks"; "We found that there was a clear": "Southern California University Professor's Study," *Ascribe News*, April 4, 2006.

p. 115: "Exercising would be the best thing": "The Physical and Psychological Benefits of Walking," HealthNewsDigest.com, April 24, 2006.

p. 126: "review published in the *American Journal of Psychiatry*": Robert Golden et al., "The Efficacy of Light Therapy in the Treatment of Mood Disorders: A Review and Meta-analysis of the Evidence," *American Journal of Psychiatry*, April 2005.

Chapter 5: The Happiness Diet

p. 133: "Inflammation appears to be": Janet Cromley, "Diet Sometimes Steps in Where Drugs Won't Tread," *Vancouver Sun*, June 7, 2008.

p. 134: "The data from randomized studies": Joseph Hibbeln, "From Homicide to Happiness," Cleave Award Lecture, 2007.

p. 134: "Many nutrition experts believe": Andrew Weil, "Ask Dr. Weil: Fatty Acids Confusion Takes Some Sorting Out," *Vancouver Sun*, May 7, 2007.

p. 136: "Studying thirty-eight different nations": Joseph Hibbeln et al., "Healthy Intakes of n-3 and n-6 Fatty Acids: Estimations Considering Worldwide Diversity," *American Journal of Clinical Nutrition* 83, 2006.

p. 138: "an increased risk": Joseph Hibbeln et al., "Maternal Seafood Consumption in Pregnancy and Neurodevelopmental Outcomes in Childhood," *Lancet*, February 17, 2007.

Chapter 6: A Journey of the Soul

p. 143: "Happiness comes from the health of the soul": Stevenson, *The Home Book of Proverbs*, p. 1069.

p. 146: "Nowhere nor in anything": Leo Tolstoy, *The Kingdom of God Is Within You: Christianity Not as a Mystic Religion But as a New Theory of Life* (London: William Heinemann, 1894), p. 80.

p. 146: "One expert defined religion": Harold Koenig, "Spirituality and Depression: A Look at the Evidence," *Southern Medical Journal,* July 2007.

p. 146: "The religion of the future": Connie Schultz, "Searching for Enlightenment, Americans Adapt Buddhism," *Plain Dealer* (Cleveland), April 11, 1999.

p. 147: "A variety of religions": Amy A. Kass, *The Perfect Gift: The Philanthropic Imagination in Poetry and Prose* (Bloomington, Ind.: Indiana University Press, 2002), p. 407.

p. 147: "I am a Hindu. I am a Muslim": "Gandhi's Legacy Betrayed," *Al Aahram Weekly On-line,* October 3, 2002.

p. 148: "The truth is that you are always united": Clive Johnson, *Vedanta: An Anthology of Hindu Scripture, Commentary and Poetry* (New York: Harper & Row, 1971), p. 34.

p. 149: "people with high levels": Michael McCullough, David Larson, "Religion and Depression: A Review of the Literature," *Twin Research,* June 1999.

p. 149: "Religion produces positive effects": Michael Argyle, *The Psychology of Happiness* (New York: Routledge, 2001).

p. 149: "Dr. David Larson . . . found a strong pattern": Stephen Kliewer, "Allowing Spirituality into the Healing Process," *Journal of Family Practice,* August 1, 2004.

p. 150: "When we know what the ends": Julia Annas, *The Morality of Happiness* (New York: Oxford University Press, 1995), p. 109.

p. 151: "Every single night": Daniel Chanan Matt, *The Zohar: Pritzker Edition* (Palo Alto, Calif.: Stanford University Press, 2003), p. 204.

p. 152: "Hard it is to understand": Paul Carus, *The Gospel of Buddha: Compiled from Ancient Records* (Chicago: Open Court Publishing Co., 1915), pp. 75, 76.

p. 153: "Whatever joy there is": Donald S. Lopez, Steven C. Rockefeller, *The Christ and the Bodhisattva* (Middlebury College Symposium Papers) (Albany, N.Y.: SUNY Press, 1987), p. 81.

p. 153: "Be they Muslims, Jews": Thomas F. Cleary, *The Essential Koran: The Heart of Islam: An Introductory Selection of Readings from the Qur'an* (New York: HarperCollins, 1994), p. 9.

p. 153: "Anyone, male or female": Ibid., p. 39.

p. 154: "Absolutely, God's allies"; "This is the true triumph": *Quran: The Final Testament: Authorized English Version, with the Arabic Text*, Rashad Khalifa, trans. (Universal Unity, 2001), p. 168.

p. 154: "You have no idea how much joy": Ibid., p. 337.

p. 154: "Now the man of perfect virtue": Miles Menander Dawson, *The Ethics of Confucius* (New York: Cosimo, 2005), p. 122.

p. 154: "Those who are not looking": John Templeton, *Wisdom from World Religions: Pathways Toward Heaven on Earth* (West Conshohocken, Penn.: Templeton Foundation Press, 2002), p. 273.

p. 154: "The blessed holy one revealed": Matt, *The Zohar*, p. 392.

p. 155: "a strong correlation exists": S. G. Post, "Altruism, Happiness, and Health: It's Good to Be Good," *International Journal of Behavioral Medicine* 12, 2005.

Chapter 7: Living Well Emotionally Well-Being Program

p. 161: "Just being alive, having a wonderful family": "The Things They Wrote," *New York Times*, March 24, 2004. The soldier was later killed in action a few weeks after writing this letter in September 2003.

p. 163: "The Gospel of Thomas": John Dart, *Unearthing the Lost Words of Jesus: the Discovery and Text of the Gospel of Thomas* (Seastone, 1998), *passim*. Excerpts from the Gospel of Thomas: the Gnostic Society Library, the Nag Hammadi Library, the Gospel of Thomas, translated by Stephen Patterson and Marvin Meyer, http://www.gnosis.org/naghamm/gosthom.html.

p. 164: "Gratitude is at the core": Anita Curtis, "C'mon, Get Happy," *Dallas Morning News*, November 10, 2007.

p. 164: "Life is available only": Thich Nhat Hanh, *Peace Begins Here: Palestinians and Israelis Listening to Each Other* (Berkeley, Calif.: Parallax Press, 2004), p. 23.

p. 164: "He who binds himself": William Blake, *Poems & Prophecies* (Read Books, 2006), p. 383.

p. 164: "The greatest thing is to give thanks": Robert A. Emmons,

Thanks! How the New Science of Gratitude Can Make You Happier (New York: Houghton Mifflin, 2007), p. 26.

p. 165: "Research from my laboratory": *The Today Show*, NBC, January 16, 2006.

p. 165: "Pay attention"; "It's a joy": Barbara Hey, "Paths of Peace: The Wisdom of Thich Nhat Hanh," *Better Nutrition*, March 2003.

p. 165: "You may recognize": Thich Nhat Hanh, *Taming the Tiger Within: Meditations on Transforming Difficult Emotions* (New York: Riverhead Books, 2004), p. 205.

p. 165: "Please take a pen": Ibid., p. 189.

p. 166: "Every moment is an opportunity": Thich Nhat Hanh, *The Heart of the Buddha's Teaching: Transforming Suffering Into Peace, Joy & Liberation* (New York: Broadway Books, 1999), P. 177.

p. 166: "Each minute, each second": Thich Nhat Hanh, Arnold Kotler, *Peace Is Every Step: The Path of Mindfulness in Everyday Life* (New York: Bantam Books, 1992), p. 26.

p. 168: The concepts of "Three Good Things," "Gratitude Journals," "Gratitude Visits," and "Signature Strengths" was written about in detail by Martin Seligman, Tracy Steen, Nansook Park, and Christopher Peterson in "Positive Psychology Progress: Empirical Validation of Interventions," *American Psychologist*, July–August 2005.

p. 168: "to extract the maximum": Lyubomirsky, *The How of Happiness*, p. 92.

p. 168: "People keeping gratitude journals": Curtis, "C'mon, Get Happy."

p. 169: "There's a natural tendency": Stacey Colino, "Do You Have What It Takes to Be Happy?" *Shape*, May 2005.

p. 171: "The remarkable thing": Wallis, "The New Science of Happiness."

p. 172: "Be an experiential epicure": Daniel Goleman, "The Secret of Happiness: It's in the Genes," *Austin American-Statesman*, July 21, 1996.

p. 173: "There is one factor": "The Pursuit of Happiness," *Allure*, February 2007.

p. 190: According to Dr. Richard Rosenthal, a newer form of MAOI antidepressant, selegiline (Emsam), is delivered in a patch form and doesn't have the same dietary restrictions as the oral form.

About the Authors

Montel Williams is an Emmy Award–winning talk show host, a decorated former naval intelligence officer, entrepreneur, motivational speaker, and philanthropist. He is the author of the *New York Times* bestsellers *Living Well; Climbing Higher;* and *Mountain, Get Out of My Way,* and the coauthor of the *New York Times* bestseller *BODYChange.*

In 2006 Montel became National Spokesperson for the Partnership for Prescription Assistance, a major industry campaign to extend prescription drug help to all Americans. In 2008, the PPA celebrated giving prescription assistance to its five millionth person.

Prior to hosting his own television show for seventeen years, Montel was a special duty intelligence officer in the navy, specializing in cryptology. A graduate of the Naval Academy, he received a number of military awards and citations during his naval career. Before attending the Academy, he enlisted in the Marine Corps after graduating from a Baltimore, Maryland–area high school.

In 2005, he was named chairman of the National Veterans Association (NVA) and has taped public service announcements for both the NVA and the Paralyzed Veterans of America (PVA).

Montel has worked with an array of charitable organizations, including the Make-A-Wish Foundation, the Joey DiPaolo AIDS Foundation, and the Humane Society of the United States. Currently, he serves on the boards of the We Are Family Foundation, devoted to promoting tolerance and diversity through educational programs aimed at the youth of America; the PVA; and The Montel Williams MS Foundation.

In 1999, Montel announced his diagnosis with MS, a potentially debilitating autoimmune disease that affects the brain and spinal cord. To raise both awareness and funds for MS research, he created The Montel Williams MS Foundation.

William Doyle is an award-winning writer based in New York, and the bestselling coauthor with Montel Williams of *Living Well*.

24.95

158 W
Williams, Montel.
Living Well Emotionally.